There Is

LIFE

After

BREAST CANCER

There Is
LIFE
After
BREAST CANCER

ATTIE DE VRIES

CREATION HOUSE
A STRANG COMPANY

THERE IS LIFE AFTER BREAST CANCER by Attie De Vries
Published by Creation House
A Strang Company
600 Rinehart Road
Lake Mary, Florida 32746
www.creationhouse.com

This book is not intended to provide medical advice or to take the place of medical advice and treatment from your personal physician. Readers are advised to consult their own doctors or other qualified health professionals regarding the treatment of their medical problems. Neither the publisher nor the author takes any responsibility for any possible consequences from following the information in this book.

Cover design by Terry Clifton

Library of Congress Control Number: 2006936891
International Standard Book Number: 978-1-59979-153-1

First Edition

07 08 09 10 11— 987654321
Printed in the United States of America

*I dedicate this book to the
women in my life:*

*My sister, Tina Infranca;
My daughters, Jacqueline De Vries,
Yvonne Brock, Wiete De Vries, and
Bonnie De Vries;
And my precious granddaughter,
Christina Brock.*

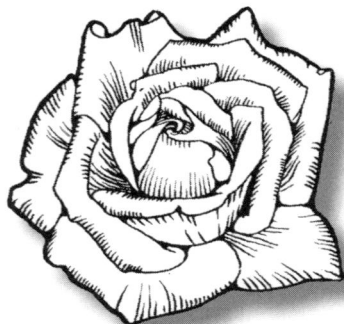

Acknowledgments

I THANK GOD FIRST of all for helping me to write this book. For without God this book would not have been possible.

My mom, who has gone to be with the Lord, for her courage when she was facing brain surgery, and her trust in the Lord. She has been an example to me.

My husband Simen, who after I shared with him about writing this book encouraged me and said, "Let me pray for you, that the Lord will help you," and as he finished praying, I got up and wrote the outline and most of the book in about two weeks, one year after my second brain surgery. He continually encouraged and prayed for me.

To Kathi Macias for her encouragement and for proofreading the book and putting the dots and commas in the right places.

To my daughter Yvonne, who read the book, believed in it, prayed for me, and put the periods and commas where they should be. She listened to me and gave me some helpful suggestions as I shared the book with her.

Jacqueline, our oldest daughter, who prayed for me and made sure that everyone she came in contact with prayed for her mom.

I thank Simon and Michael, our sons, and my daughters-in-law Wiete and Bonnie, who prayed faithfully for me, and helped me when I needed help to learn the computer, so this book could be written they were there to help me.

My brothers Jan and Hanke, and sister Tina, for their prayers, support, and being there as I went through the surgeries.

To Doctor Schemmer, the staff of St. Jude's Hospital in Fullerton, California; Dr. Steven Giannotta and the staff at the University of Southern California (USC) Medical Center in Los Angeles; and Dawn Fishback, Physicians Assistant at USC University Hospital Neurosurgery, for being so patient in answering all the questions I had. Thank you all, for everything you have done.

Contents

Introduction

EVERY YEAR, TWO hundred forty thousand women will be diagnosed with breast cancer, and nearly forty-six thousand women will die of the disease. That is why it is so important to take yearly mammograms. For, early detection, not procrastination, can save lives. Cancer found early can be 100 percent curable.

I was diagnosed in 1995 with breast cancer, and again in 2001 with two brain tumors. I am a survivor, and I give God all the praise for this. It is my prayer that as I share my journey of cancer with you, it will be an encouragement to you.

Cancer does not have to be a death sentence. I am living proof of that.

> For I know the thoughts that I think toward you, says the Lord, thoughts of peace and not of evil to give you a future and a hope.
> —JEREMIAH 29:11

God has made each of us
special and unique. No one
else has our DNA blueprint.

I will praise You,
for I am fearfully and
wonderfully made.
— Psalm 139:14, NKJV

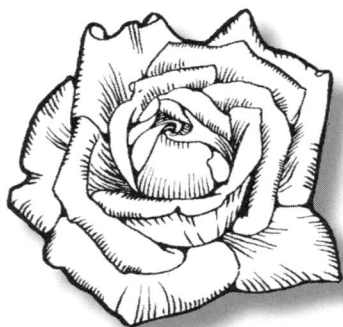

Chapter 1

We Found a Nodule

THE TELEPHONE WAS ringing—nothing unusual. It seems that our phone rings a lot at dinnertime.

My brother was visiting from Holland and staying at my mom's home, so we invited them over for dinner. I had prepared a special candlelight meal. Everything was cozy, the conversation pleasant, and then the phone rang. *Not again,* I thought. *Why does this always happen at dinnertime? Probably just another phone solicitor.*

I took the phone into the office so as not to disturb the mealtime conversation. "Mrs. De Vries," I heard on the other line, "this is Doctor All."

Dr. All? I thought. *Why is she calling me?* There was a pause before she explained.

"I went over your mammogram today, and we found a nodule in your right breast. Can you come in tomorrow? I want a closer look at this just to be sure. It probably is fine, but just to be safe we will retake the mammogram and some close-ups."

"What time shall I come in?" I asked.

"Is ten o'clock all right for you?"

"Sure," I said. "I will be there."

"Good," she said, and with that she hung up.

I sat at my desk for a minute, not knowing what to think about this conversation. Just that morning, I had a routine mammogram, but thought nothing of it. I returned to the dinner table, stunned at this turn of events. Other than a slight pain under my right arm, I had been feeling fine—until now.

"Who was that on the phone, At?" my husband asked. When I explained about the nodule and my need to go in the next day for a closer look, there was silence around the table. Our conversation had suddenly taken a turn from recalling the past to being plopped down smack in the middle of life with all its problems. It was as if we had just dropped a bomb in the middle of a pleasant evening.

"Well," my husband said, "I will go with you tomorrow." The conversation was over, leaving me alone with my doubts, concerns, and questions.

I Knew I Needed a Mammogram

Just one month before, I read an article in a Christian magazine about the actress, Ann Jillian, who was a survivor of breast cancer.[1] What got my attention as I read, was that for some time I had had a pain under my right arm. It did not seem to be anything serious, but reading her story made me think that maybe I should have a checkup and a mammogram. I closed the magazine and tried to forget it, but I could not.

I have always heard that you are to have a mammogram every year after the age of forty, and I was over forty. I began to wonder to myself, *when was the last time I had a mammogram? Have I ever had a mammogram?* I could not remember. Is it an X-ray? In fact, I was so ignorant about what a mammogram actually was, I came to the conclusion that I never had one.

I remembered that my doctor had told me to have a mammogram five years earlier, but I ignored her advice. So when I read Ann Jillian's success story about breast cancer, I was again reminded of my need for a mammogram.[2] As a result, I made an appointment at the Women's Health Center, but I could not get in until October.

I shared with them that our youngest son, Michael, was getting married in Holland and I would not be back in the U.S. for another four weeks, so could they somehow squeeze me in before I left for Europe? They could not. But in the meantime, the doctor wanted me to take hormone pills or the "hormone patch" which were good for my bones at my age she said. The hormone patch is a Vivelle-Dot estrogen patch, similar to the pill, only now you do not have to remember to take your pill each day. It automatically releases the hormones into your body on a daily basis. They also suggested I try to get an appointment for a mammogram at the hospital. But they didn't have any openings until October. I therefore decided not to take the suggested pills or the "hormone patch" until I got back from Europe and had my mammogram. I later learned how lucky I was for not taking these drugs.

We soon left for Holland to attend the wedding of our son to a beautiful Dutch girl, Wiete. My husband and I are originally from Friesland, Holland. When you look at the map of Europe, you will see this tiny country in the upper left corner of the map, next to Belgium and Germany. If you look even closer up in the northern part of Holland, you see Friesland. I was born in Leeuwarden, which is the capital city of Friesland. If you drive from the airport, Schiphol, to Alkmaar to Den Helder, you go over a big dike in the middle of the sea, called the Afsluit dike. Once you drive through this, you arrive at a town called Leeuwarden. It has an atmosphere all its own— back in time.

~~~~~~

At the age of seven, I gave my heart to the Lord at the Salvation Army. In 1952 I met my husband, Simen, at a ballroom dance on a Saturday evening. As my husband explained later, he saw these two cute girls walking in front of him. He said to his friend, "Wherever those two are going, we go. You take the red-haired girl, and I'll take the dark-haired girl," which happened to be me. I was fifteen and Simen was eighteen. We discovered that we lived around the corner from each other.

As I found out later, Simen had big plans for the future. He wanted to go to America, and he asked me how I felt about that. I had mixed emotions about it; what about my family? It was not an easy decision to make; but then, I did not have to make it yet. We were so young, and besides, Simen had to go into the Dutch air force for two years when I met him. *A lot can change in that time,*

I thought. Simen and I went steady for four years before he emigrated to America. I followed one year later, with all the excitement one feels when one is twenty-years-old, and going overseas to a land that promises a glorious future. Life was full of adventure. Four weeks after I arrived in America, we were married in a Dutch Christian Reformed Church service in Pasadena, California. We started a family and the Lord blessed us with four children, two boys, Simon and Michael, and two girls, Jacqueline and Yvonne.

It was exceptionally nice for us to see our son getting married in our native country to such a nice girl. We knew her parents, Bert and Willy Dorenbos, long before we knew our daughter-in-law. Every time we were in Holland we saw each other and had dinner together. The first time I met Wiete was when she was about sixteen, in Switzerland, when we attended "The European Religious Broadcasters" conference about fourteen years ago. We sat down for dinner at the hotel where we were staying, when Wiete asked if she could join us for dinner. I remember thinking, *What a nice girl—potential daughter-in-law? You never know, if we ever get her to the U.S.* Years later, her father suggested that maybe Wiete should visit us in California. I thought it was a great idea. She came, met our son Michael, and the rest is history.

Before you knew it, we were on our way to the wedding in Holland, along with the whole family. It was quite a celebration! We had a lot of fun while we were there. We had dinner together, and all our grown-up children and some of their friends attended the wedding, as well as aunts and uncles from the U.S., and others still living in Holland. It was quite an affair, as weddings in Holland are all-day events.

Early in the morning, the groom arrived at the house of the bride to take her to the church for the ceremony. Simen performed the wedding ceremony, and Wiete's dad did the message, taken from Proverbs 3:5–6:

> Trust in the Lord with all your heart, and lean not on your own understanding; In all your ways acknowledge Him, and He shall direct your paths.

God has a plan for our lives and He will direct our lives if we ask Him. If we rely on our own ability or wisdom, we will fail. But if we ask the Lord, He will guide us. Our understanding is limited; we can only know and see so far. But the Lord knows the future. He sees the beginning and the end.

It was a great message not only for the newlyweds, but for all of us. After the church service, we all went to the Van der Valk Hotel in Hilversum for entertainment, a skit by the Dorenbos family, good food, coffee, and especially a *gebakje*, a wonderful Dutch treat.

Finally, the time came that we all had to go home, and that meant making an appointment with the doctor. I am always amazed at how quickly we adjust to another way of life, after leaving Europe and returning home to the everyday life we left behind for a little while. With so much to do upon returning home, there was a temptation to let my appointment go. But thankfully, I didn't. I had the mammogram done, and then came the phone call.

I Am Not Every Woman

The next day, when I went in for some additional pictures, I was somewhat surprised by how many they took. After I thought we were finally finished, the nurse showed up again and said, "Mrs. De Vries, we need one more picture."

"Why?" I asked.

"The doctor wants some close-ups so he can look at it more closely," she answered, and with that she walked out of the room. Soon she returned with additional slides. "One more," she said, "and then you will be ready to go." I never thought I would have so many pictures taken of my breast!

After we finished, the nurse instructed me not to get dressed until the doctor had seen the film. "Wait until I come back, and then I will tell you when you can go," she said. Finally, she returned. "You are done," she said. "You can go now." She handed me a pink flower, which I thought was nice.

At the front desk, I asked if I could have a copy of my mammogram. "If you call your doctor, she will provide you with a copy," I was told. "We cannot give it to you." The next day was my appointment with my doctor, who again explained to me that there was a nodule in my breast. Then she told me she wanted me to see a breast surgeon named Dr. Kenneth Schemmer. She handed me his telephone number and said, "Call him."

"May I have a copy of my mammogram?" I asked.

"Sure, I will have the girl in the office run off a copy for you. I hope everything will turn out all right for you," she said, as she left the room.

Simen and I decided we would go out for lunch, as we had a lot to talk about. As we walked out of the room, the girl in the front office said, "Mrs. De Vries, here is your medical report." We went to our family's favorite restaurant. Simen ordered our lunch, and I was deeply intrigued reading my medical report. In essence it said, "The findings on the mammogram are not cystic and, as described on the mammogram, most likely represent that of a *focal ductal ectasia.*"

As I read, I said to my husband, "How can they know that? I'm not a doctor, but as far as I can tell, unless you take a biopsy, how will you know what it is?" We talked and talked, and I said, "I really want to be sure of this diagnosis. It is too important. Let's go back to the radiology department, Simen, and ask them some questions. How did they arrive at this conclusion?"

When we arrived at the radiology department, we asked the girl behind the desk if there was someone I could speak with about my report. "The doctor who dictated your report is in," she said. "I will ask if he can speak with you."

We waited for about five minutes, and then the girl came back and told us the doctor would see me. After a short greeting with the doctor, I handed him my report.

He looked at it, and then I asked him, "How did you come to the conclusion that this is probably a *ductal ectasia*? Don't you have to do a biopsy first before you can know exactly what it is?"

His reply frankly startled me. "Well, ma'am," he said, "we can't do a biopsy on every woman who comes in here with a nodule in her breast." My face must have shown disbelief, because he went on in great length to explain, that many women have lumps in their breasts at some time in their life. The cause could be too much coffee or tea; in short, too much caffeine. He said if they did a biopsy on every woman with a nodule they would be in surgery all day!

I was somewhat taken back by his nonchalant approach. I thought, *I am not "every woman." I have a nodule in my breast, and I want to find out what it is. I don't care about statistics of "every woman."*

Though we had not learned much more about my condition, I left with the understanding that I had to be in charge of my health, not the doctor. The next day I made an appointment with the surgeon for Thursday afternoon at two o'clock. I was instructed to bring all my records with me.

You have a choice: find out if it is
cancer, or whatever comes will come.

Before every man there lies a
wide and pleasant road that seems
right but ends in death.

–Proverbs 14:12, TLB

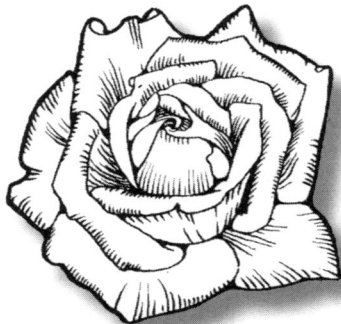

Chapter 2

Early Detection Saves Lives

D R. SCHEMMER WAS the breast surgeon. His office was a pleasant place, airy, light, and friendly, with a nice girl working at the front desk. I felt comfortable right away.

"Mrs. De Vries?" The girl smiled as she looked at me. When I nodded, she said, "Follow me." With that she opened the door into another waiting room. "The doctor will be right with you," she said. Simen and I sat down, quietly caught up in our own thoughts, as he held my hand. Finally, the door opened, and the surgeon walked in.

"Congratulations, Mrs. De Vries," he said. "I've been reading your medical report, and you are fine!"

Stunned, I asked, "Did you read my mammogram? I have a nodule in my breast!"

"Yes, I read it," he said, "but I am sure it is harmless. I am 99.9 percent sure you have no cancer."

I looked at him in disbelief. "Can you guarantee this 100 percent?" The doctor looked at me, smiled, and said,

"No, only God can do that. But, in my opinion, I think you can wait six months and then take another mammogram."

"What then?" I asked. "What are we going to do if the nodule is still there?"

"We do a biopsy," he answered.

"I prefer a biopsy now," I said. "I don't want to wait six months. I would rather be safe than sorry."

"If that is the way you feel," the doctor said, "we will schedule you for surgery."

Early Detection—Not Procrastination— Saves Lives!

For some time, I thought that it was just my doctor who advised me to wait six months before doing a biopsy. But, to my amazement, I learned that quite a few doctors say that to their patients. Many women have told me the same story, though I am happy to say, not all women listened to their doctors and insisted on doing a biopsy immediately. At the same time there are too many who wait, and live in the false security of what they don't know won't hurt them. Many wait even longer than six months to follow up. You have two choices: you either find out what it is, or you say, "Whatever comes will come."

A friend of mine decided she was going to wait and lost her life one year later. Another friend commented, "You have to believe your doctor, At!" The problem with that is that too many women want an excuse for not finding out. They think, *What if I have cancer? I don't want to know*. When I was talking recently to a young woman who discovered a lump in her breast, she looked at me and said, "Sure I'll see a doctor, I'll promise!" After some months went by, I asked her "Did you ever find out about the lump in your breast?" To my amazement, she said, "No, but I will." I don't know if she ever found out. Another woman said to me, the doctor said I have nothing to worry about it is only a "cyst," she did not question the doctor, she later told me, because this is what she wanted to hear. Later, when through a set of circumstances she found out she had breast cancer, she said, "What if? What if?"

Fear can lead to poor judgment, wrong choices and decisions.

> There is a way which seems right to a man and appears straight before him, but at the end of it is the way of death.
> —PROVERBS 14:12, AMP

Early detection can save a life—your life! Cancer *in situ* is 100 percent curable. It refers to tumors that have not grown beyond the site of origin, into neighboring tissue. This is good news, and is the reason why early detection is so important. Procrastination can mean a less favorable outcome. Having a mammogram is so easy; maybe a little uncomfortable, but not painful.

So don't be anxious about tomorrow.
God will take care of your tomorrows
too. Live one day at a time.

—*Matthew 6:34, NLT*

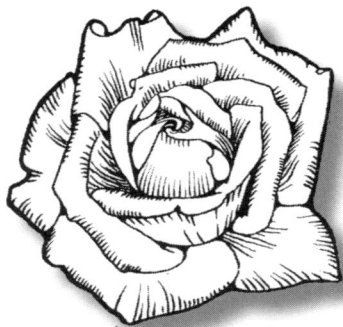

Chapter 3

The Biopsy

THE LONG-AWAITED DAY of the surgery came, and we arrived at the hospital at six in the morning. The girl at the counter knew why we were there and handed me some papers to fill out. Our daughters, Yvonne and Wiete, arrived just before my surgery to offer moral support. "We will pray for you, Mom, during surgery," they assured me.

"Mrs. De Vries," the nurse said as she opened the door. "Come on in. We will start in about fifteen minutes."

After a quick "I love you" to my family, I was transported into the unknown. As I entered the room, I saw a large mammography machine in the middle of the room. The nurse was busy with all kinds of needles, small ones and larger ones.

"You can get undressed now," the nurse said, and handed me a blue coat. "Leave it open in the front, and I will be right back."

I looked around the room as I put on the robe, and wondered, *What are they going to do?* There was a knock on the door, "May we come in?" asked the nurse. With her was a doctor. We exchanged a brief hello, and then they went to work. Pictures were taken under the guidance of the doctor, as they needed to find the exact spot for the needle to enter for the biopsy. This explained the need for all those needles on the table.

The nurse prepared a solution and said, "This will sting a little, but it's nothing to worry about, Mrs. De Vries." As she turned to get the needle, I saw the size of it and said, "Is he going to numb the area before he puts that big needle in my breast?"

"No," she said, "but it really will not hurt that much. It will only sting." As she handed the needle over to the doctor, she must have seen my apprehension because she said, "Stay very quiet, Mrs. De Vries. We will be done very quickly." Later, I found out that she should have numbed the spot! After all this preparation was over, they allowed the family to stay with me until I was wheeled into surgery.

"Mom, you'll never believe who is going to do your surgery," our daughter-in-law, Wiete, said.

"Yes, I met him last week," I said.

"I know, but guess what? Doctor Schemmer was in Holland last year visiting my parents, and I met him there." Wiete's parents have a ministry called Cry For Life. Dr. Schemmer had gone to Holland to meet with some of the European doctors who are interested in abolishing the euthanasia law. He wrote a book on the subject called, *Tinkering With People.*

What a small world! I thought. I was delighted to learn that not only had our daughter met him, but also that he was a born-again believer. I knew I was in good hands.

The Lord knew I was there, the doctor was a believer, and I felt blessed. After we all held hands and prayed, I was wheeled into the operating room. When I got there, I looked around at all the nurses and doctors, and I thanked the Lord for their help and dedication.

I had been transported into a different world, a world we normally do not think about when we are healthy. The Lord sure uses these men and women to bring healing and comfort to so many families in need when we ask Him, for all healing comes from God. As the doctor finished the surgery, he still had to wait for God to do the healing.

When I am in a hospital and I see families waiting for their loved ones to come out of surgery, I realize how important it is for us to hold them up in prayer. What a blessing to pray for our loved ones and the medical personnel asking God to bless and give them guidance and wisdom! It was some years ago that a physical therapist said to me, "I noticed that children who are prayed for do better than the ones who are receiving no prayer." Yet she herself was not a Christian; she merely observed this.

The surgery went well. At 8:30 a.m., Dr. Schemmer came into the waiting room.

"Can you tell us anything?" my husband asked.

"No, not yet," the doctor replied. "In about three days we should know." In the meantime they wheeled me into the recovery room, sleepy but fine. Simen was the first one to see me. "Hi, honey," he said. "How are you doing?"

"All right," I whispered, smiling. "What did the doctor say, Simen? Was it cancer?"

"We won't know for a couple of days, Attie." Frankly, I was prepared if it was cancer.

"You want a cup of coffee, Mrs. De Vries?" the nurse asked.

"Please," I said. "That would be great!" I had nothing to eat or drink for hours, and a cup of coffee sounded great.

We all went home soon after, and then we waited and talked. I wondered to myself, *What if it was cancer?* There was a real possibility of that, we knew. I wanted to be prepared, and had been reading about breast cancer and all the options women have these days. It is a world you never think about if you are not faced with it.

I Will Trust God

The waiting was the most difficult. I am a take-charge kind of person; I see what needs to be done and do it. I like to organize and get going, but this time I had to wait. There was nothing else I could do. My thoughts went back some thirty years ago, to an older couple in our church. Their ministry was to encourage the young people and pray for them. Simen and I had been the recipients of their prayers and encouragement. There was something special about them they were so peaceful, nothing seemed to upset them.

When I went through a very difficult time in my life, it was that couple who prayed for me. I remember them saying that we have to trust the Lord, and that not our will, but the Lord's will be done (author's paraphrase; see Luke 22:42).

I listened, but did not really grasp it, until five years later when I was at the lowest point in my life, and I am sure it was Jesus who brought this couple to my remembrance who knew the Lord when I did not. Oh, I had accepted Jesus as my personal Savior, and I had peace with the Lord, but I did not know Him in a personal way, because I did not acknowledge Him as Lord over my life. I did not even know how to trust or love God, and I was sure those people did. There was something about them that I wanted. There was a peace that I wanted; they trusted God.

That morning, I cried out to the Lord, and I said, "God, I want to know you." No more playing around, going to church, coming in the same way as going out. I wanted to know God. I wanted Him to help me, just like He did our friends. And you know what? The Lord touched me! It was as if I got a present that morning. No one was around. I was sitting at the kitchen table wondering, *What is life all about?*

I realized something was wrong with my relationship with the Lord. I had major problems and no peace with Him. I instinctively knew that if I said I was a Christian, then I should trust the Lord. *What is wrong with me?* I wondered. Our friends had that inner peace, and I wanted it.

When the Lord touched me that morning, it was the beginning of a new life for me. It was as if someone had given me a present. Not everything was solved that day, but I started to walk with the Lord. I talked to God about everything and I have never been the same since. That was about thirty-five years ago.

Over all those years, the Lord did a work in my life. "being confident of this very thing, that He who has begun a good work in you will complete it until the day of Jesus Christ" (Phil. 1:6, NKJV). The Lord works it in, and we work it out. It is all a work of God if we dare to yield ourselves to the Lord and trust Him in everything.

Life can be demanding. We live in a society that demands all of our time. Many of us feel as if we have no time for ourselves. So many demands come our way, that only what is important to us will be done. We have to prioritize our lives—what is important to us, or better yet, who is important in our lives.

Jesus says, "And you shall love the Lord your God with all your heart, and with all your soul, with all your mind, and with all your strength" (Mark 12:30, NKJV). It is a way of life. "Your heart," means God communicates His Word to our hearts. He puts His searchlight on our heart, "For the eyes of the Lord run to and fro throughout the whole earth to show Himself strong on behalf of those whose heart is loyal to Him" (2 Chron. 16:9, NKJV). And, "you shall teach them diligently to your children, and shall talk of them when you sit in your house, when you walk by the way, when you lie down, and when you rise up" (Deut. 6:7, NKJV).

When you are born again, God communicates with us in our spirits and He will let us know His plan for our lives. We can talk to God about everything and He will hear us. We walk not by our own desires, but by every word that proceeds from God. He will guide us by His peace. When the Lord speaks to us, we will have a peace in our heart when we obey Him. Do we love God first? Do we seek Him first in our lives? If we do, then the Lord will take care of us. That is why Jesus says, "But seek first the kingdom of God and His righteousness, and all these things shall be added to you" (Matt. 6:33, NKJV).

The problem is whether we believe that. Or, do we only think about it, but pretend to believe it? Jesus says, "For whoever desires to save his life will lose it, but whoever loses his life for My sake will find it" (Matt. 16:25, NKJV). We say, "I will it and I will find it." Wrong! Acknowledge God in all your ways and He will direct your path.

We live in a Me society, where everything is geared to pleasure. It is very much the now generation. What about our children? Are we an example for our children? Do we lead them to Jesus? Many young people do not know why they are here, or what God's purpose is for their lives. God has a plan and purpose for all of our lives.

We cannot go wrong if we give our lives over to the Lord, because He made us—shouldn't He know what is best for us? There is a song that says it all:

> Have Thine own way, Lord! Have Thine own way!
> Thou art the Potter, I am the clay.
> Mold me and make me after Thy will,
> While I am waiting, yielded, and still.
> Have Thine own way, Lord! Have Thine own way!

Hold o'er my being absolute sway!
Fill with Thy Spirit 'till all see
Christ only, always, living in me.[1]

Many times, as I walk in the California sunlight, I am so thankful to the Lord for who He is, for my husband and children and grandchildren, for where we live, for our home. There are many times that I say, "Thank You, thank You, Lord, for the privilege of knowing You, and for all that You have done!" What a blessed people we are; the enjoyment of being alive to enjoy every moment of it is wonderful! *Will I still be grateful for everything when I found out the news I was about to receive?*

The Lord admonishes us to not, "Be anxious for nothing, but in everything by prayer and supplication, with thanksgiving, let your requests be made known to God; and the peace of God, which surpasses all understanding, will guard your hearts and minds through Christ Jesus" (Phil. 4:6–7, NKJV).

Then, and only then, will we experience God's peace. This peace does not depend on how we feel, what news we just received, how much money we have, who we are, but on who God is! He is the Giver of life. He is the all-knowing God. Nothing is a surprise to Him. The Lord is faithful. If we keep our minds and thoughts focused on Him, He will keep us in His perfect peace.

I am eternally grateful to the Lord for everything, in the good days, and also in the not so good days. The day I received the news of my cancer was, as you might guess, one of the not so good days, yet I felt the peace of God as I listened in on the phone conversation.

Oh, put God to the test and see how
kind He is! See for yourself the
way His mercies shower down on
all who trust in Him.

−Psalm 34:8, TLB

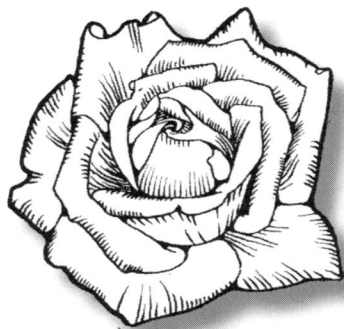

Chapter 4

It Is Cancer

THE PHONE RANG, and my husband picked it up. "This is Dr. Schemmer and we have the results of your wife's biopsy. It is cancer. I would like you and your wife to come into my office tomorrow to discuss the options for surgery." My husband looked over at me, and said, "Sure, we will be there." We looked at each other as my husband got off the phone, and I knew.

We then discussed what the doctor had said. I was prepared! I was sure that God would help us and see us through this time in my life, no matter what the outcome. I experienced firsthand what the Lord had done in my life. This was not me. I knew who I was. Jesus was the One who gave me this peace in my heart.

Faced with cancer, it was not terrifying for me. God had worked a trust in my inner being that was amazing to me. I faced cancer, even death, and yet I could still say, "I will trust God no matter what the outcome will be." I truly had come a long way! Only the Lord can work that in a person's inner being, when we give ourselves over to Him.

When our son was incurably sick some thirty years ago with scleroderma, I wrote a book about it. I was a different person then, and faced with losing our son, I was about to give up on life when the Lord touched me. As I knelt next to our bed, crying out to the Lord, I was aware of His presence. I felt the love of God that evening. He spoke to my heart and asked, *Why is it so difficult for you to give him over to me? I love him far more than you will ever love him.* When I realized the love of God for our son, for me, and for all of us, it was easy to give him over to the Lord. All the turmoil left and there was peace in my heart! For the first time in many months, I was able to give our son over to the Lord and say, "Not my will, but Your will be done." No more taking back; just leaving him in God's hands. It felt like a weight had been lifted off my shoulders, and the burden was gone. It was God who had worked this in me; I knew I could never have done it. When faced with cancer in my own life, I experienced that same peace of knowing that God is in control.

You never will know what is in your heart until you face difficulties. Where do you go but to the Lord? It is He who gives us the strength for the occasion.

Sweet Willing Surrender

Actress Ann Jillian described the role faith played in her life by telling the story of a memorable visit to church shortly before her mastectomy.[1] As she was leaving the church that day, she saw an inscription on the outside of the building: "The same everlasting Father that looks after you today will look after you tomorrow and every day. Either He will shield you from suffering or He will give you the unfailing strength to bear it."[2]

Ann described feeling dumbfounded. She recalled that the inscription was exactly the message she needed to hear. Instead of quitting in the face of this adversity, she decided to surrender, not to the disease, but to God.

"I am going to fight this thing," she said to God. "But ultimately, do with me as You will."

"That's the ultimate surrender," Ann said, "sweet willing surrender to God's work, knowing and trusting fully in Him that whatever He has in His beautiful hand for us is the true and right thing to do. "That was the moment of growing up," she concluded. "That was the moment of success."[3]

All that God wants from us is that we trust Him. It is that simple.

⁓

The next day, Dr. Schemmer explained the different procedures: lumpectomy with radiation, or a mastectomy and no radiation.

"What about a lumpectomy and no radiation?" I asked.

"No," he responded. "If you do not want radiation, then I advise you to do a mastectomy."

"What about chemo?" I asked.

"We don't know yet until we have all the results in," he said. "We'll know a lot more after the surgery. Hopefully there is no lymph node involvement, so let's wait and see, and then I will go over everything with the both of you. In the meantime, you let me know if you prefer a mastectomy or a lumpectomy and radiation. It is my opinion that a lumpectomy with radiation is just as good as a mastectomy, but you decide."

Going home we had a lot to think about and, above all, to pray about. That morning I was reading about King Solomon, the son of King David. When King David passed away his son became King and he realized he needed help. That is a good place to be—"God please tell me what to do!"

God appeared to him in a dream that night and told him to ask for anything he wanted, and it would be given to him! Solomon replied, "You were wonderfully kind to my father David because he was honest and true and faithful to you, and obeyed your commands. And you have continued your kindness to him by giving him a son to succeed him. O Lord my God, now you have made me the King instead of my father David, but I am as a little child who doesn't know his way around. And here I am around your own chosen people, a nation so great that there are almost too many people to count! Give me an understanding mind, so that I can govern your people well and know the difference between what is right and what is wrong. For who by himself is able to carry such a heavy responsibility?" (1 Kings 3:6–9).

The Lord was pleased with his reply and was glad that Solomon had asked for wisdom, "So he replied, 'Because you have asked for wisdom in governing my people and haven't asked for a long life, or riches for yourself, or the defeat of your enemies—yes, I'll give you what you asked for! I will give you a wiser mind than anyone else has ever had or ever will have! And I will also give you what you didn't ask for-riches and honor! And no one in all the world will be as rich and famous as you for the rest of your life! And I will give you a long life if you follow me and obey my laws as your father David did'" (1 King 3:11–14, TLB).

Whether it be King Solomon or a mom who is just diagnosed with breast cancer, we all need wisdom. Nothing is too big or small for the Lord, He will give wisdom to whom ever will ask. I loved that story in God's Word. It really touched me.

God has a plan for our lives. If we rely on our own ability or wisdom, we will fail. But if we ask God, as King Solomon did, God will give us wisdom.

Talking it over with our family was hilarious! My mother who was eighty-three years old, said, "I have never heard of anything like this. You want to remove your breast?"

"But, Mom, I have breast cancer," I explained.

"Yes, but remove your breast? Oh yeah, yeah! What is this world coming to!" she responded.

Another family member asked, "Are you kidding? You do not have your breasts chopped off!"

My husband said, "You pray and think this through then you decide."

I did pray for wisdom, and I asked the Lord what is the right thing to do. *How much more advice?* I prayed, *How many more opinions do I get?*

29

Ultimately it depended on what I was comfortable with. The doctor had given me some options and I had a choice. It is not like twenty years ago, when women went into surgery for a biopsy and, if they found cancer, the breast was totally removed. Today, they send you home and you have time to make a rational decision. But the doctor did caution me after he saw my reluctance about radiation, "If you do not want radiation, then have a mastectomy."

So I was left to make a decision that with God's help only I could make. Surgery was scheduled for February 1995. Doctor Schemmer had spoken to me briefly a couple of days before surgery, saying, "Let me know what you want me to do, and we will do it." The day before surgery I decided to trust God for the doctor's wisdom.

I called the office and told the receptionist to tell Dr. Schemmer that I would trust his judgment on what to do. He was doing the surgery, and I believed that the Lord would guide him either to perform a lumpectomy or a mastectomy. I believed that when the doctor performed the surgery, he would know if the cancer was confined or if it had spread. He would be better able than I to make the right decision. I left it in the hand of the surgeon, believing that God would direct him. Both the surgeon and his assistant were believers in the Lord.

Where do you put your trust?
In man? In your
circumstances? Or in God?

For God has not given us a spirit of
fear, but of power and of love and
of a sound mind.

–2 Timothy 1:7, NKJV

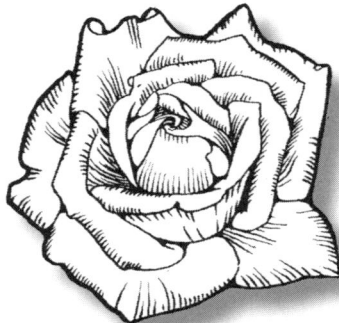

Chapter 5

Faith Versus Fear

THE FIRST TIME I heard the word *cancer* was in Europe during World War II. Our neighbor was diagnosed with cancer. We did not know too much about the disease then, except that it was a somewhat mysterious disease. People were fearful about it. Today we are more informed and talk more openly about it. We raise money for resources to find a cure. We have support groups for cancer patients and their families. Everyone is, in some way, touched by it, or knows someone who has cancer.

But, for many people, cancer is a real shocker; "The Big C," as it is sometimes called. That Big C is better understood when we substitute Christ the Healer, the great Physician. Doctors can only do so much, but God does all the healings.

We may as well ask ourselves these questions, "Where does our focus lie? In whom do we put our trust: man or God? Or in our circumstances?" God wants to bless you more than you want to receive it, for nothing is impossible with the Lord.

There is a story in the Book of Numbers in chapters 13 and 14 that illustrate what I am trying to say, which I will paraphrase. When Moses sent twelve spies into the Promised Land, ten came back saying, "We were like grasshoppers in our own sight There are giants in the land! Does God want us to be killed?" they asked. They expressed fear. All they saw were giants. Joshua and Caleb had a good report, and said, "The land we passed through to spy out is an exceedingly good land. If God delights in us, then He will bring us into this land and give it to us. Do not fear the people!"

But they did not listen. The majority of the people believed the ten spies who gave a fearful report. All they saw were obstacles. We can put our trust in God or we can look at our circumstances and give up.

What are your giants? Each of us at one time or another in our lifetime will face a situation that will require what we believe. Do we believe God or do we put our trust in what we see? Fear destroyed their spiritual inheritance. God wanted to give them the Promised Land, but because of fear they lost out. Many people are fearful of the unknown, and of failure, man, death, and of cancer. If we let fear take over, it will rob us of a blessing.

> For I am persuaded that neither death nor life, nor angels nor principalities nor powers, nor things present nor things to come, nor height nor depth, nor any other created thing, shall be able to separate us from the love of God which is in Christ Jesus our Lord.
>
> —Romans 8:38–39, nkjv

Betsie, the sister of Corrie ten Boom, a Holocaust survivor, said, "There is no pit so deep that God's love is not deeper still."[1] So true, if we can but grasp this truth.

A friend of mine was diagnosed with breast cancer ten years ago, and in the course of a conversation we had, she said, "I still wake up every morning with the thought, 'I have breast cancer.'" So, I posed this question to her, "Do you think this is the Lord?"

"No of course not," she said. After ten years of being cancer free, she was still afraid.

"Well," I said to her, "let's go through this. You know it is not the Lord, and you also know it is not a fact, because you are cancer free."

"Yes," she answered.

"Well, then, the only alternative left is the devil. He stands every morning at your bedside and scares you. He is the author of fear! He is the one who puts you in bondage," I continued.

I shared with her some of the principles of resisting the enemy, "Therefore submit to God. Resist the devil and he will flee from you" (James 4:7, NKJV). It is wonderful if you can find a friend who you can share your fears with. For in doing so, the enemy is exposed and when exposed you can take a stand and command him to go and he will flee from you. When we submit to the Lord, we then free ourselves for God to work in our lives. He can heal us, or He can use the physician and go through it with us, and give us the peace of mind and strength we need. Something good will always come out of the situation for those who love the Lord, "And we know that all things work together for good to those who love God, to those who are called according to His purpose" (Rom. 8:28, NKJV).

Me writing this book and encouraging you is a miracle. Only the Lord is able to do this, so be encouraged, because I am a breast cancer survivor.

⚬

When I received word that it was cancer, there was a peace that only the Lord can give, a peace that passes all understanding. In fact, I was even pleasantly surprised. You never know your reaction until you are faced with it, and then you understand what is in your heart.

What I found out was this: even when the news was not good, I still enjoyed the California sun, my family, my home, and above all, I love God and trust Him in everything in the good days and in the not so good days! Why, you might ask. Well, simply because God is God, He does not miss a thing! He is all-knowing. There is a purpose in everything. God did not look down on us and say to His angels, *Oh, we forgot Attie! Now she has breast cancer, because we overlooked her.* No, the Lord knows everything. He does not make us sick. Jesus says, "The thief does not come except to steal, and to kill, and to destroy. I have come that they may have life, and that they may have it more abundantly" (John 10:10, NKJV).

Do I understand it all? No, but I don't have to, and I trust the Lord. I am totally dependant on the Lord for everything, and I still have the peace to enjoy life to the fullest. Not only that but I had the privilege to write a book on breast cancer and to be an encouragement to someone else, by saying, "You can make it with God's help." I feel blessed to know the Lord, to be able to take what seemed a disaster and use it for good; the devil might have meant it for bad, but the Lord will use it for good.

It is not so much of what happens to us in life, but what are we doing with it that counts. Life can be an adventure. Every day is a new day, a new beginning.

My prayer is that you might find the Lord and that you might find a more fulfilled life, and as you wake up every morning you will thank and praise the One who made you, for He alone can give you a real purpose in life. Life can be an adventure, and every day will be a new beginning. As you wake up in the morning, praise God for another day, and ask Him to help you.

Fear not, for I am with you.
Do not be dismayed.
I am your God.
I will strengthen you;
I will help you;
I will uphold you with
my victorious right hand.

—Isaiah 41:10, TLB

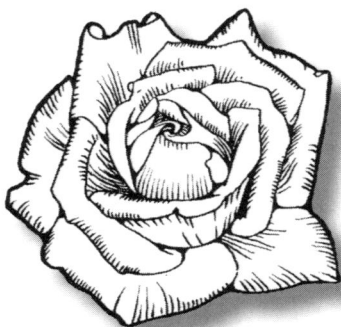

Chapter 6

Surgery

I WAS VERY FORTUNATE to have my family with me. They where a great support system.

When my daughter-in-law heard I was diagnosed with breast cancer, she came over after work and said, "Mom, let's go shopping tomorrow. I will take you wherever you want to go. You want to go to the bookstore? Have dinner? Do some shopping? Whatever you want, we will do." That really touched me. She was, and is, so sweet.

When faced with surgery, the prospect of needing blood is a possibility. It is an excellent idea to donate your own blood, or get some from trusted family members. The hospital will give you a couple of days, or a week, before surgery, but you have to let them know that you prefer your own blood. Mistakes are made if you, or a member of your family, are not watching it.

I became aware of this some years ago when my husband needed blood before surgery. We had given blood for him, believing he would receive it when he needed it. But I found out that you have to follow the blood and make sure it will be given to the right person.

In the surgery room and in the intensive care room is a refrigerator with the donor's blood. I was visiting my husband in intensive care, when the doctor ordered the nurse to give my husband some blood. I watched her as she walked to the refrigerator, took out a pint of blood, and put it on the bed before she gave it to him. I looked at the label and read it. "This is not our blood," I said to the nurse, "You took the wrong blood."

"Sorry," was her reply, and with that she changed the blood for my husband's blood. From that moment on whenever we give blood we make sure only our blood will be given. Do not leave it to chance! Make sure your name is on the bag. That is why you gave it—it is for you!

The evening before surgery, we came together as a family to talk and pray. It was difficult for our grown-up children to express their fears. I tried to help them by sharing my feelings about cancer and told them that the Lord would see us through. Suddenly one of our children started to cry. "I am afraid, Mom, that you will die," he said. We all had tears in our eyes as we freely expressed our fears that evening. We all prayed as a family, not only for me, but also for our family that the Lord would give them peace, for the doctors and nurses, and for God's healing touch.

As I looked around the living room, I felt so blessed to see our children and my mother looking to the Lord for help. That alone was such a blessing! As we finished praying I said, "I will be fine. God will see us through!"

The day of the surgery arrived, and we anticipated a good outcome. Surgery was scheduled for six a.m. As

I arrived at the hospital, there were more papers to fill out. It always amazes me how much paperwork there is. As I was ushered into the surgery prep room, a nurse handed me a gown. "Put this gown on and tie it in the back," she said. "And I have a bag for you so you can put all your other belongings into it." After I did what she told me to do, I hopped in bed to wait for what was next.

The nurse came in with a doctor whom I had not met, and the anesthesiologist, who wanted to know my whole medical history. After he was through, my family came in and we all prayed, and asked the Lord to be with me and with all the doctors and nurses. Then off I went. My prayer was, "God, my life is in your hands."

The surgery took about two hours, and the whole family was waiting when finally the doors opened and Dr. Schemmer came out with a thumbs up! "Your wife is doing great," he said. "She tolerated the surgery well, and it looks like we got it all. It looked very clean, so we decided to do a lumpectomy, but she does need radiation afterwards. We will have the results of the lymph nodes in a couple of days."

Simen thanked the doctor, and then all of them thanked the Lord, for His mercy. To celebrate, everyone decided to have lunch, including Dad and all our grown-up children and their spouses, my mother, my brother, and sister. But before they went out to eat, they strolled in to take a peek at me, one by one. I was still very sleepy, and Mom tried to feed me too many ice chips at the time. It was because I complained to them about a dry mouth, so Mom had tried to help.

"Attie needs her rest, so let's all go out to lunch," my husband suggested. Later on I heard how much fun they had!

My mom even bought a new dress for the occasion. We were shopping together a week before my surgery when she saw this dress she wanted to buy. "But, Mom," I protested, "this dress is too big for you!"

"Did you see how much they lowered the price, Attie? It's on sale!" she said.

I tried to talk her out of it. "Mom, this dress does not fit you," I said. "It's at least two dress sizes too big!"

"But I like this dress," she said. "And did you see how much money they took off the dress? It's a bargain, At!"

"I give up. You want the dress, go and buy it," I said, hoping she would hang the dress in the closet and forget about it. But she did not, as I heard later. Mom was set in her ways; once she had made up her mind about something there was no talking her out of it. My brother had no idea what he was in for that day of my surgery. Mom came a half hour later with my brother, who had to drive her to the hospital. They were both staying at our home.

Mom decided she was going to put on her new dress for this special occasion. "Go ahead," my brother said. "I'll wait for you." When they were ready to go, my brother looked at the dress and said, "Are you going in that dress? It's too big on you!" He continued, "No way, Mom, do I go out with you like that. That dress does not fit you! We cannot go unless you put on a dress that fits you."

Mom took one look at him and said she was going! With that she went to the kitchen and handed him a pair of scissors. "Here," she said, as she handed the scissors to him, "cut the dress."

"How do you want me to cut this dress?" my brother asked, knowing he was going to lose the battle.

"Well," she said, "just cut all around me and make it shorter." She was sitting down and refused to stand up, so he only could cut the front of the dress.

When they finally came walking into the hospital, Mom's dress was cut uneven, with a big train in the back, and everyone laughed!

"Mom, what happened?" they asked.

"Hanke cut my dress," she said. They all had to inspect her dress as my brother tried to explain what had taken place at home. They all had a good laugh. Mom's dress was short in the front and long in the back, like a wedding dress. It was hilarious!

When you are eighty-three, life is simple. Mom enjoyed lunch with her family, and she knew I was fine. That was all that mattered.

After all those years we still have a laugh about it. I had breast cancer surgery, and Oma (Mom) came in with an uneven dress. It sure broke the tension that day!

If you want to know what God wants
you to do, ask Him, and He will
gladly tell you, for He is always
ready to give a bountiful supply of
wisdom to all who ask Him;
He will not resent it.

– James 1:5, TLB

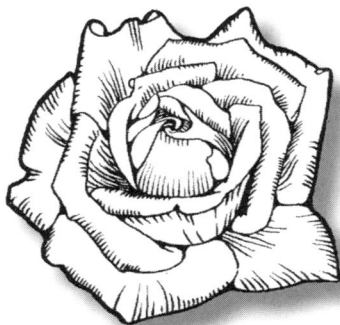

Chapter 7

Decisions, Decisions

As I woke up from surgery, the first thing I did was place my hand over my right breast.

What happened? I wondered. *No mastectomy? I still have my breast?* At first, I was somewhat disappointed. I looked up at my husband, who was sitting next to my bed, and asked, "What is going on, Simen? I still have my breast!"

"Well, honey," he explained, "everything looked so clean, that the surgeon decided a lumpectomy was fine. Plus, of course, you will need radiation. Just try to rest, and we will talk later."

With that I dozed off into never-never land. Later that afternoon I was able to go home. The recovery was easy. The difficult part was not able to dress myself. I also had a drain at the side of my breast to remove fluid that can collect around the incision in the armpit. The drain is actually a soft plastic tube that travels from your arm pit, down along your side, to a small bulb at your waist, which the doctor removes in about a week or so. The doctor also prescribed painkillers if needed.

My husband was a great help, and I could recuperate in leisure. The children are all grown up and married, so I did not have to take care of them. That is one plus as you get older.

Our next appointment was a week later. We discussed radiation in about four weeks. We also talked about the drug Tamoxifen or chemotherapy, which we would decide on when all the test reports were in.

It gave me plenty of time to research what I wanted to do. I prayed about it, listened to the doctors, and read about the different options available. Some books were very helpful, and I have included a list of them at the end of this book.

There are women who, when diagnosed with breast cancer, prefer a total mastectomy, while other women want a lumpectomy. Depending on your individual history, you can make an intelligent decision. Then there are women who do not like radiation, or Tamoxifen, and prefer to go the natural health food way, meaning no drugs or radiation. Tamoxifen, as I see it, has its pros or cons. There are many decisions to be made, things to think about, and a lot to read. I personally did not have a difficult time deciding on a lumpectomy or a mastectomy, as either was fine. My worth as a woman does not depend on whether I still have my breast. I was more inclined not to have radiation, though I do not really know why. Maybe it was somewhat mysterious.

Radiation

As we entered into the radiation department, a nurse met us.

"I have an appointment to see the doctor," I said.

"Yes, we are expecting you, Mrs. De Vries. Just follow me." With that she took us to the doctor's office. He introduced himself to us and said, "Take a seat and I will explain the procedure." We sat down and he said, "Today, radiation therapy is almost always recommended as a follow-up to lumpectomy, to eliminate any cancer cells that might remain. Researchers consistently find that radiotherapy is highly effective in preventing local recurrences. Local recurrences may be 25 to 30 percent higher among women who do not receive radiation after a lumpectomy. Side effects do occur, such as scarring of the lungs, but in time that will most likely heal. The good news is that it is painless."

He must have seen the apprehension on my face because he said, "Let me take you through our facilities, and you can see for yourselves."

It was a quiet day; we were the only people there. As I walked into the radiation department and saw the huge machine I felt uneasy. First I contributed it to the unknown. Radiation, it just does not sound good; it has somewhat of a mysterious ring to it. All I ever heard about radiation was that it kills people. We all have heard about Chernobyl in Russia, where one of the reactors failed, causing many fatalities and sickness to overexposure of radiation. How, then can this be good for me?

47

The doctor tried to put me at ease. Before we went to this place, I had told my husband that I only wanted to see first; I did not know yet if I was going through with this. The doctor had a different idea.

"We can give you your first dose of radiation right now," he said. "All you have to do is lay on this table and the machine will do the work. It goes around your body for a few minutes, and then it is over. We will do this procedure every day for six weeks. Toward the end we will give a boost dosage, it is another type of radiation delivered directly to the spot where the cancer was."

It all went a little too fast for me. I thought we had only made an appointment to see the doctor and discuss the procedure, and perhaps set a future time for me to come in, so I would have time to think about it.

"We have an opening today," he said "just take it; once you go through it, you will be fine."

I looked at him and thought, *Maybe he's right*. That day I got my first dose of radiation treatment, which took less than a minute. Blood tests were also taken, just as a precaution, to check the red and white blood cells. In the middle of my treatments, three weeks into it, I developed a rash, or "hives" as the doctor explained. I wondered if it was due to the radiation. No one knew for sure.

Because of this problem, I wound up in the emergency room twice. Consequently, the radiation was stopped for three or four days. Then we resumed the treatments again. Everyone was puzzled about why this had happened. When the six weeks were over, I visited my oncologist, who noticed extreme tenderness in the radiated breast.

"How long has this been going on?" he asked.

"Since the radiation treatments," I said. I thought this was normal and that every woman experienced this after radiation.

"No," he said. "This is somewhat unusual. I have never seen it this tender. I will send you to a specialist."

The appointment was made for the next day. After examining me, the doctor said, "Let's do a biopsy and see what is going on." The following week, a biopsy was performed and the report came back as "chronic inflammation" and "dermal fibrosis," and no trace of cancer, which was good news. I felt I should have followed my instinct, and paid attention to my reluctance about receiving radiation. It did not mean however, that this is also for you, because radiation might be a good thing. For me, it brought some problems.

The doctors were puzzled and said, "We don't know. This is a rare case." One doctor did admit that he had seen more problems because of radiation; what those problems were he did not say. For me, I can only say, go by your instinct; pray about it, and if you feel good about this, go for it. There are many women who do well with radiation. But before you agree to radiation, check around. There is a steady improvement in radiation therapy for cancer, including three-dimensional or stereoactive radiation, ultra high-speed radiation, and proton-beam radiation. Much of this information can be found on the Internet. Your typical radiologist might not know about it. It is up to you to find out; it is your health we are talking about.

You might not need to be exposed to unnecessary radiation. Some doctors may not know these diagnostic tools. They might not read up on it or go to these informative seminars. But on the other side of the coin, Solomon, the wise King, had this to say about too much information, "And further, my son [daughter], be admonished by these. Of making many books there is no end, and much study is wearisome to the flesh. Let us hear the conclusion of the whole matter" (Eccles. 12:12, NKJV). Meaning, when all is said and done, there is only one thing that really matters, and that is this: "Let us hear the conclusion of the whole matter: Fear God and keep His commandments, for this is man's all. For God will bring every work into judgment, including every secret thing, whether good or evil" (Eccl. 12:13–14, NKJV).

Pathology Report

Always ask for a copy of your surgery and pathology reports as most doctors are happy to give them to you. Occasionally, a doctor will make a comment like, "Let me worry about your health; you do not have to." The doctor should worry about my health instead of me? I don't think so. Who, more than I, will follow up on my health? It is my experience that doctors are too busy to worry about my health.

Chemo

In some instances, chemotherapy is considered. Not all women are the same; each one is different, with different needs. Make sure you have your pathology report with you when you go to your oncology doctor. There are alternative treatments available, but you have to do the research on your own. The key is not to be passive, but be aggressive when it comes to your health for that matter, your loved ones health.

Ask yourself, what do you think about the treatment offered to you? Are you okay with what they want to do? Or do you want to explore other alternatives and be in charge of your own health? I, personally, am amazed when I meet women who have been diagnosed with cancer and they cannot tell you what kind of cancer, how large the tumor is, or even what is going to take place next. Be informed! Knowledge is power! And above all, ask the Lord to help you and to give you wisdom in what approach to take.

Tamoxifen

I was offered Tamoxifen, also known by its brand name Nolvadex. It has been used since 1974. I did not feel comfortable with taking this drug after I did some research on these drugs used for cancer. A study is out now that every woman who is at risk for breast cancer can now take this drug Tamoxifen. The theory is that it can prevent breast cancer in high risk women.[1] As for me, I did not take this drug, but as I stated before, you have to do your own research on it.

Tamoxifen is most often used following a lumpectomy and radiation treatment in post-menopausal women who are hormone positive [ER, RR]. If your estrogen receptors are negative, Tamoxifen is unlikely to work.[2] Chemo will most likely be offered, though it depends on the individual woman.

I was a good candidate for Tamoxifen because my test came back as hormone positive receptors. But after doing some research on the pros and cons of this drug, I found there is a risk of blood clots, which carries the same risk when taking birth control pills. Also, you have a five times greater risk of getting endometrium cancer, the same as women taking estrogen replacement therapy.[3] You're better off taking estrogen replacement obtained in your local health-food store.

As for me, I stay away from Tamoxifen. I was not convinced this drug was good for me. Pray about all your decisions. Ask the Lord for wisdom, and He will give it to you!

DNA Analysis

This test tells you how aggressive your cancer is. The normal complement of DNA is found in the nucleus of a cell. If it tells you it is a diploid, the cancer might be less aggressive. If on the other hand the cancer cell contains less or more than a normal amount of DNA, it is called an "aneuploid," meaning the cancer is more aggressive. The DNA index for a diploid cancer is 1.00. Any number higher or lower than that indicates an aneuploid tumor.[4]

Grades

Grades look at the pattern of a tumor cell and nuclei. It signifies how aggressive the cancer is. Grade 111 the most aggressive, while grade 1 is the least.[5] You want to know all this and more before you make a decision on how to approach your treatment. Ask your doctor, who, after all knows all about the treatment that will best work for you.

It was once believed that only older women have breast cancer, but now we find that even women in their early twenties can get it. Also, women are at a higher risk if a family member, a mother or a sister, develops the disease.

USC Norris Comprehensive Cancer Center has announced the opening of a clinical trial, evaluating intra-operative radiotherapy following lumpectomy for the management of early stage invasive breast cancer. Eligible patients will be randomized to receive single dose intraoperative radiotherapy given at the time of lumpectomy or conventional post-operative radiotherapy given daily for a six- to seven-week period. The ultimate goal of the trial is to improve the convenience and feasibility of breast conservation by allowing women to complete surgery and radiotherapy in a single day.[6]

There is also a new study out, "SonoCiné," a computer-guided ultrasound. Mammography misses 50 percent of all cancers in dense breast tissue and up to 25 percent of all breast cancers. "SonoCiné is an investigational method of whole breast ultrasound undergoing a multi-center trial to determine if breast screening by ultrasound can discover breast cancers not found by Screening Mammography or physical examination."[7] In the back of this book you will find a website where you can find more information on this study.

True, 80 percent of women have a benign nodule. But thousands are among the 20 percent whose biopsy will read breast cancer. When you read the pathology report of your biopsy for the first time, you might be some what puzzled. What does this mean? Ask questions, read up on it, or go to the Internet, where you can find a wealth of information.

A biopsy report will tell you if you have cancer, or if it is a benign condition such as fibrocystic changes or a fibro-adenoma.

The pathology of a cyst also can identify an abnormal cell of atypical or an excessive cell growth of hyperplasic or atypical hyperplasic. The last one puts women at a higher risk of breast cancer. It all takes a biopsy to find out for sure.

And if it is cancer, what kind is it? Is it a ductal carcinoma, or is it lobular carcinoma, or is it both, which is called an adenocarcinoma. If the cancer is confined in the duct, it is called or classified as an *in situ* or intraductal carcinoma which is 100 percent curable. But once it leaks out, it is a different story. It is then called invasive or infiltrating breast cancer.[8]

Paget's disease of the nipple is a very rare breast cancer, which resembles a rash, somewhat like eczema. Inflammatory breast cancer is characterized by swelling, redness, and warmth, and diagnosed by a skin biopsy. Invasive ductal or lobular carcinoma, is also called infiltrating ductal or lobular carcinoma, meaning the cancer has spread from its original site in a duct or lobule and has started to grow into surrounding tissues. Invasive ductal breast cancer is the most common, accounting for about 75 percent of all breast cancers.[9]

Finding the cancer early can be a lifesaver! Cancer in situ is 100 percent curable. Therefore, early detection is a must. Read your mammogram report, and when a nodule is discovered, do not wait six months or longer. Have it taken care of. Why wait?

In the *Orange County Register* there was a report about a study done that favored a magnetic resonance imaging test (MRI) for high-risk women.[10] The new research claims that twice as many tumors are found with an MRI than with an ordinary mammogram. Researchers studied 1,909 Dutch women, including 358 with one of the BRCA genes or other mutations that predispose women to breast cancer. Up to half of such women get it by the time they're fifty and are prone to ovarian cancer. "Women who are at high risk should consider getting MRI besides mammography," said Dr. Stephen Feig, a radiology professor at Mount Sinai in New York.[11] There are many more options for early detection. Cancer does not have to be a death sentence. Therefore early detection saves lives!

A friend of mine died of breast cancer at the age of fifty-one. The sad part is that she knew for one year that she had a nodule in her breast, and yet she refused to see a doctor until it was too late.

In talking to many women I found out that she is not an isolated case. Fear of taking a mammogram, fear of a biopsy, not wanting to know the truth, holds many women back. We should face our fears and not run from them.

The Bible says that people are destroyed for a lack of knowledge! We would not dream of not fixing our car when it needs repair. Where do we bring our car? We take it to the most reliable auto mechanic, and we want to know what is wrong. We also ask how much it will cost. Some people even want to see the old part that was replaced so they can check if the new part was really put in. Yet, when it comes to our health many are afraid to ask questions.

It always amazes me. The same is true with our eternal destiny. Do you know where you are going after this life? If your answer is, "I do not know," or "I hope I will go to heaven. I tried to live a good life, that is all I can do," then you are wrong. We can never be good or perfect; we all come short of the standard God has set.

You might never have gone to church or you may have been in church all of your life and yet, not know Jesus. But the good news is that Jesus paid the price for our sins. "For God loved the world so much that he gave his only Son so that anyone who believes in him shall not perish but have eternal life" (John 3:16, TLB).

All we have to do is recognize that we are in need of forgiveness for our sins. We cannot earn it. It was paid in full when Jesus died for our sins on the cross. It is the grace of God that saves us. We will never live without sin as long as we live on this earth! We need the forgiveness of our sins through the blood that was shed on Calvary for whosoever will.

"For all have sinned and fall short of the glory of God" (Rom. 3:23, NKJV). And, "If we confess our sins, He is faithful and just to forgive us our sins and to cleanse us from all unrighteousness" (1 John 1:9, NKJV). Galatians 2:20 says, "I have been crucified with Christ: and I myself no longer live, but Christ lives in me. And the real life I now have within this body is a result of my trusting in the Son of God, who loved me and gave himself for me" (TLB).

If you have never asked the Lord into your life, then let me pray with you. Simply pray, *Dear God, I ask You to forgive my sins, and come into my heart. I believe You died on the cross for my sins. I am sorry, God. I give You my life, in Jesus name, amen.*

When you pray this prayer and meant it, then Jesus promises to give you eternal life, and you will never lose it. Now you have eternal life through out the ages. Life eternal, what a blessing! You can freely and boldly come before God and talk to Him, and He will hear you. Talk to the Lord about everything. Ask the Lord to heal you, to be with you and He will!

You have two choices.
You can go introspective in a
negative and fearful way, or you
can face cancer and take a stand!

Jesus says, "The thief's purpose is
to steal, kill, and destroy.
My purpose is to give life
in all its fullness."

–John 10:10, TLB

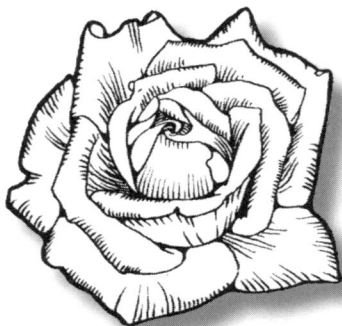

Chapter 8

What Good Can Come Out of Cancer?

WHAT GOOD CAN come out of cancer, you might ask? Well for one thing, it will let us look at our lives in a different perspective. What are we doing? Where are we going? It can be a blessing if we let it be. It can open our spiritual eyes and allow us to see life in a different light. A verse comes to mind that says, "For what profit is it to a man if he gains the whole world, and loses his own soul? Or what will a man give in exchange for his soul?"(Matt. 16:26, NKJV).

We have a choice we either will go introspective in a negative and fearful way, or we will rise to the occasion and make the most of it with the help of the Lord. In other words, we can become more productive and wiser in more than one way. The good news is that with God all things are possible!

Cancer does not have to be a death sentence. The Lord is still on His throne, even when we are diagnosed with cancer. God still heals people, who seemingly should not have made it. He is still the same, "Jesus Christ is the same yesterday, today, and forever" (Heb. 13:8, TLB). The Lord has the last say in how long we are going to live. There are people who received news that they had only six months to live and are living still ten years later, much to the amazement of the medical profession. It is because the Lord healed them!

We can also leave a legacy for our children. Tell them it is a wonderful thing to be alive! If a person lives to be very old, let him rejoice in every day life, but let him also remember that eternity is far longer, and that everything down here is futile in comparison.

> Young man, it's wonderful to be young! Enjoy every minute of it! Do all you want to; take in everything, but realize that you must account to God for everything you do.
> —ECCLESIASTES 11:9, TLB

I love the Book of Ecclesiastes. The writer is Solomon, son of King David. Solomon was a wise man, who said, "I have seen it all!" (Eccles. 1:2, author's paraphrase). Did you ever say or think that? I have, or feel I have, or I have asked, "Now have I seen it all?" Well, Solomon did, and this was his conclusion, "Vanity, Vanity! All is Vanity" (Eccles. 1:2, NKJV). He says, "Here is my final conclusion: fear God and obey his commandments, for this is the entire duty of man. For God will judge us for everything we do, including every hidden thing, good or bad" (Eccles. 12:13–14, TLB). Every person who has ever lived— a solemn thought indeed!

We Tend to Pray More

Prayer changes things. Years ago a friend invited me to a Bible study on prayer and it changed my life. It was a simple Bible study with some everyday illustrations of how we can come to God with everything. How we can hear the voice of God. In essence, she explained that praying is just talking to Jesus, and believing that He hears and answers our prayer. God is interested in the everyday affairs in our lives! It revolutionized my life that day.

Prayer is putting in action what God wants us to do. Jesus says, "For I have come down from heaven, not to do My own will, but the will of Him who sent Me" (John 6:38, NKJV). When we pray in the will of God and are open to His will for our lives, God will put in our hearts what we should pray for. "Now this is the confidence that we have in Him, that if we ask anything according to His will, He hears us. And if we know that He hears us, whatever we ask, we know that we have the petitions that we have asked of Him" (1 John 5:14–15, NKJV). Sadly, most people pray more when in trouble. When all goes well in life and they are busy, there is a tendency to forget to talk to God on a daily basis. But the minute we face difficulties we run to the Lord, "Where our help comes from." Listening to this Bible teacher I learned one simple thing "you can talk to God about everything!"

Just prior to that experience I had rededicated my life to God, saying "If you are there I want to know You." I was all by myself that morning, the radio was on and

I heard a minister say, "You can talk to God." It was as if I had received a present, there was a expectancy that God will hear me. It was only a couple of days later that I attended the Bible study.

How can God talk to you? Or, better yet, how do I hear from God? God does not have the problem, we do. We have trouble listening and hearing. What is it that you want me to do God? We seem to have a problem listening to the voice of God, and when we do know what to do, of obeying the Lord. There is a song that says it all: "Trust and obey, for there's no other way."[1] In a nutshell, that is it. Simple, yet so true. Trust and obey.

One young woman confessed to me that she believed the Lord was telling her to have a "talk fast," which meant to stop talking and start listening more to what God was telling her. So true! It is difficult for many people to sit still long enough to hear. If we will just read the Bible every day, talk to the Lord, and listen to His voice and obey Him, we will be blessed indeed. In a nutshell, nothing is too small or too big for the Lord!

I still remember her from that Bible study class some thirty years ago saying, "When I drive down the street and I get lost, I call on God for directions and He helps me." I realized how the Lord is interested in our every day lives. *Well,* I thought, *if God speaks to her, He will speak to me.* And right there in that church I asked the Lord to talk to me. It was a simple Bible study, yet so profound. So basic, yet so difficult for most of us to understand; that the God of the universe is interested in our everyday life, that we can come to Him in prayer and talk to God about all of our problems.

I always went out from the premise that I should not bother God with little things, yet I learned that day that God is interested in all of our affairs. He never sleeps nor slumbers. We are the problem, not God. As a matter of fact, Jesus has a lot to say in how we ought to pray. He started with, "Our Father in heaven, we honor your holy name. We ask that your kingdom will come now. May your will be done here on earth, just as it is in heaven. Give us our food again today, as usual, and forgive us our sins, just as we have forgiven those who have sinned against us. Don't bring us into temptation, but deliver us from the Evil One. Amen" (Matt. 6:9–15, TLB).

"Our Father" simply means we acknowledge Him as our Father. As we accept Jesus, His Son, who died for our sins on the cross, "For God loved the world so much that He gave his only Son so that anyone who believes in him shall not perish but have eternal life" (John 3:16, TLB). We need to be born again. There is a wonderful story of one man's encounter with the living God found in the Book of Acts.

Paul and Silas were in jail. And around midnight they were praying and singing hymns to the Lord, and the other prisoners were listening. Suddenly there was a great earthquake. The prison was shaken to its foundations, all the doors flew open and the chains of every prisoner fell off! The jailer wakened to see the prison doors wide open, and assuming the prisoners had escaped, he drew his sword to kill himself. But Paul yelled to him, "Don't do it! We are all here!" (Acts 16:28).

Trembling with fear, the jailer called for lights and ran to the dungeon and fell down before Paul and Silas. He brought them out and begged them, "Sirs, what must I do to be saved?" They replied, "believe on the Lord Jesus and you will be saved, and your entire household." (See Acts 16:30–31, TLB.) The jailer had an encounter with the living God.

Which is in heaven

"You can never please God without faith, without depending on him. Anyone who wants to come to God must believe that there is a God and that he rewards those who sincerely look for him" (Heb. 11:6, TLB). Everything God does is in the realm of faith. By faith Noah built an Ark, by faith Abraham offered up his son, by faith Moses refused to be called the son of Pharaohs daughter, by faith the Israelites marched seven times around the walls of Jericho, for they believed God. (See Hebrew 11:7–17, 24–30.) Who is the recipient of faith? It is the one who, after having received a word or a promise from God, realizes it, and acts upon it as true. As Paul the Apostle says, "I believe God that it will turn out exactly as I have been told" (Acts 27:25, NASB).

We honor Your holy name

We start our praying by praising God for who He is. We should praise and glorify God with our lives for what He has done; He gave of Himself so we could live. We owe our very life to God. He is worthy of our praise. King

Solomon understood this as he built the temple for the Lord He worshiped the only true God. "Then, as all the people watched, Solomon stood before the altar of the Lord with his hands spread out toward heaven and said, 'O Lord God of Israel, there is no god like you in heaven or earth, for you are loving and kind and you keep your promises to your people if they do their best to do your will. Today you have fulfilled your promise to my father David, who was your servant'" (1 Kings 8:22–24, TLB).

I have heard your prayer

"The Lord appeared to him the second time (the first time had been at Gibeon) and said to him, 'I have heard your prayer. I have hallowed this Temple that you have built and have put my name here forever. I will constantly watch over it and rejoice in it. And if you live in honesty and truth as your father David did, always obeying me, then I will cause your descendants to be the kings of Israel forever, just as I promised your father David when I told him, "One of your sons shall always be upon the throne of Israel"'" (1 Kings 9:2–5, TLB).

In Revelation, we see another scene of praising the Lord, the apostle John was taken up in heaven and he lets us see a glimpse of what is going on in heaven, he saw living beings all around the throne, "Day after day and night after night they kept on saying, 'Holy, holy, holy, Lord God Almighty the One who was, and is, and is to come.' And when the Living Beings gave glory and honor and thanks to the One sitting on the throne, Who lives forever and ever, the twenty-four Elders fell down before Him and worshiped Him, the Eternal Living One, and cast their crowns before the throne, singing, 'O Lord, You are worthy to receive the glory and the honor and the power, for You have created all things. They were created and called into being by Your act of will'" (Rev. 4:8–11, TLB).

We will be praising the Lord in this life and the life to come. Praise releases what God needs to do in our lives. When we begin to praise the Lord, our focus turns to the Lord instead of our self. And in so doing it is easy to give our problems over to the Lord and leave them there. All our prayers should begin by praising the Lord, for He is worthy of our praises. We owe everything to the Lord.

Thy kingdom come

This means to let Christ rule and reign in our hearts. God's kingdom is available, to us now, as we repent and ask Jesus to come into our lives. The kingdom of God is not of this earth it is spiritual, "Jesus replied, 'With all the earnestness I possess I tell you this: Unless you are born again, you can never get into the Kingdom of God.' 'Born again!' exclaimed Nicodemus. 'What do you mean? How can an old man go back into his mother's womb and be born again?' Jesus replied, 'What I am telling you so earnestly is this: Unless one is born of water and the Spirit, he cannot enter the Kingdom of God'" (John 3:3–5, TLB).

Thy will be done

Jesus is our example as He was dying on the cross for us, He was obedient. "Although He was a Son, He learned obedience from the things which He suffered"

(Heb. 5:8, NASB). Now if Jesus was obedient as the first born Son how much more should we obey the Lord in everything. "Not my will but your will be done" or "What you ought to say is, 'If the Lord wants us to, we shall live and do this or that'" (James 4:15, TLB). "Not all who sound religious are really godly people. They may refer to me as 'Lord,' but still won't get to heaven. For the decisive question is whether they obey my Father in heaven" (Matt. 7:21, TLB).

Give us this daily bread

God will provide for us everyday, this verse means more than bread, it implies that the Lord will take care of us daily. When we pray this, we, in essence, acknowledge our dependence on the Lord for everything. "So don't worry at all about having enough food and clothing. Why be like the heathen? For they take pride in all these and are deeply concerned about them. But your heavenly Father already knows perfectly well that you need them, and He will give them to you if you give Him first place in your life and live as He wants you to. So don't be anxious about tomorrow. God will take care of your tomorrow too. Live one day at a time. The righteous man shall live by faith" (Gal. 3:11, NASB).

And forgive us

"But if we confess our sins to him, he can be depended on to forgive us and to cleanse us from every wrong" (1 John 1:9, TLB). And as God forgives us, we to have to forgive. How many times, we might ask, do we have to forgive? "Then Peter came to him and asked, 'Sir, how often should I forgive a brother who sins against me? Seven times?' 'No!' Jesus replied, 'seventy times seven!'" (Matt. 18:21–22, TLB).

When we learn to forgive we set the other person free and we are free. We are no longer in bondage to that other person. Many homes are destroyed by an unwillingness to forgive. If we can just see who is behind most of the strife and difficulties in life, it is the enemy of our soul. When you read the story of Joseph, you see a glimpse of what is taking place behind the scenes. Joseph was sold into slavery by his brothers, and taken to Egypt. He was falsely accused and sent to jail.

In God's time, he came before Pharaoh. And the Lord gave Joseph the interpretation of Pharaoh's dream and as a result of this, he was put in charge, as the second man in Egypt. There was a famine in the land and Joseph was given this dream to know what to do about it. When his brothers appeared before him and recognized him they were afraid.

> But Joseph told them, "Don't be afraid of me. Am I God, to judge and punish you? As far as I am concerned, God turned into good what you meant for evil, for he brought me to this high position I have today so that I could save the lives of many people.
> —Genesis 50:19–20, TLB

It was not good what his brothers had done to him, but Joseph saw the bigger picture. He understood "That God causes all things to work together for good to those who love God, to those who are called according to His purpose" (Rom. 8:28, NASB).

Lead us not in temptation

"No temptation has overtaken you but such as is common to man; and God is faithful, who will not allow you to be tempted beyond what you are able, but with the temptation will provide the way of escape also, so that you will be able to endure it" (1 Cor. 10:13, NASB). God does not lead us into temptation, but God does permit us being tested so that we might come out stronger in what we believe. It will strengthen our faith and our character. God will make a way of escape, so take a stand! Nothing is impossible with the Lord. We can come in His presence with the smallest requests and big problems like being just diagnosed with cancer. God is in control if we surrender to Him and follow the Lord.

The kingdom and the power and the glory

God alone has the power to change a person. God alone deserves all honor and praise, "Know therefore today, and take it to your heart, that the LORD, He is God in Heaven above and on the earth below; there is no other" (Deut. 4:39, NASB). The doxology says it all:

> Praise God, from Whom all blessings flow;
> Praise Him, all creatures here below;
> Praise Him above, ye heavenly host;
> Praise Father, Son, and Holy Ghost.
> Amen.[2]

Divine surgery!

*I bless the Holy name of God with
all my heart. Yes, I will bless the
Lord and not forget the glorious
things He does for me.
He forgives all my sins,
He heals me!*

–Psalm 103:1-3, TLB

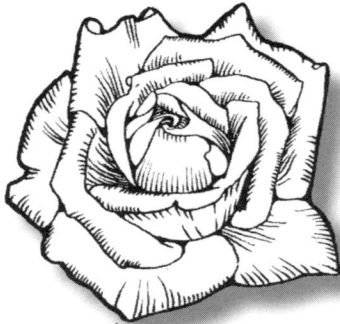

Chapter 9

A Miracle

WHEN DIAGNOSED WITH cancer, one thing will be for sure your life will never be the same. For one thing, you will have regular checkups with your oncologist, a doctor specializing in cancer. Also blood work will be done, bone scans, chest x-rays, what ever the doctor or you feel is necessary.

If another nodule is found, the question will immediately be, is it another cancer? If this happens within five years it is considered metastasis meaning the original cancer has spread. After five years it is possibly a new cancer, though not always the case. Every six months I had a checkup with the oncologist, a mammogram the first year, and after that every year a mammogram and blood test.

When I went back for my regular mammogram, not expecting to find anything different, the nurse said, "Mrs. De Vries, I need to take another picture." By then I knew this was not a good sign. When I asked if there was anything wrong, she said she didn't know but the doctor would answer my questions. Then she left the room, and I sat there wondering what was going on. I came for my usual mammogram, but this was not what I expected! For one thing, I felt fine, just as I had before my cancer surgery.

When the doctor came in, he said, "Hello, Mrs. De Vries. How are you feeling?"

"Fine," I replied. He hesitated for a moment and said, "We found another nodule in your breast."

"Another nodule," I asked. I was not expecting to hear this.

"Yes," he said. "What I am going to do is, I will set up an appointment for you tomorrow with your physician, and we take it from there." I went home, wondering what to do. When I arrived home, my husband greeted me at the door.

"Everything all right?" he asked. We sat down and I shared with him what the doctor had revealed to me.

"I will see the doctor tomorrow to see what we should do. I first want to talk to him before I make a decision, and I want to pray, to ask the Lord for wisdom."

The next day, as I was sitting at the doctor's office, I again was amazed when I looked at the faces of all the people. Even though I had been diagnosed with breast cancer once, I forgot until I was confronted with the possibility of another cancer. The nurse came to the door and called me in.

"Mrs. De Vries, follow me to room ten. The doctor will be right with you." She took my blood pressure, which was normal, as was my temperature, and she left. Then

I heard the sound of paper rustling by the door, and I knew the doctor was reading my report.

"Hello, Mrs. De Vries," he said as he walked in. "How are you?"

"Fine," I said.

"You are here because you developed another nodule in the breast?"

"Yes," I said.

"It was one year ago that you were diagnosed with cancer, true?" I nodded.

"Well, what can I do for you?" he asked, looking over his glasses at me.

"What do you suggest?" I asked, wanting to see what he had to say before I decided what approach to take.

"We can do a biopsy, and if it is cancer you can opt for a mastectomy. If it is not cancer, you're fine!"

I listened to him, knowing exactly what I wanted.

"I prefer to have a total mastectomy, this time," I said. "I do not want anymore biopsies on this radiated breast."

"Very well," he said. "I will send you to a surgeon, Dr. Schemmer, the one that did your previous surgery. And we will take it from there." He closed the file, shook my hand, and left.

Surgery was scheduled for February 1996. The evening before surgery, I asked the Lord to give me a word for that day. The next morning I woke up with a song in my heart: "For He is Lord, He is Lord! He is risen from the dead, and He is Lord. Every knee shall bow, every tongue confesses, that Jesus Christ is Lord."[1]

Simen and I were singing this song as we drove to the hospital. Our prayer was, "God, guide us today, and help the surgeons." As I was being made ready for surgery, I became somewhat uneasy about the procedure. The nurses came to wheel me into the operating room.

"Wait," they said, and put a cap on my head. When Dr. Schemmer came in, he said, "Hi, Mrs. De Vries. How are you doing?" I looked at him and started to cry. He sat on my bed, put his arm around me, and said "What is the matter?"

"I don't know," I said.

He paused, then said, "Let's take another mammogram."

"But," I protested, "I have everyone waiting for me, including you!"

"Oh," he said, "that's no problem. Don't worry about it."

They wheeled me down the corridors of the hospital to the X-ray department. Many mammograms were taken, and no nodule was found. We thanked the Lord!

When they wheeled me into the admission for the surgery room, all the nurses who had already heard the news, probably from the doctor, all clapped their hands. They were overjoyed!

Doctor Schemmer met us and said, "Mrs. De Vries, you just had divine surgery!" and then hugged me. We all thanked God and a doctor who is sensitive to the leading of the Lord! I had been only a couple of minutes away from entering the surgery room.

Why I was spared from having a complete mastectomy, yet I had to go through surgery for a lumpectomy, I do not know, but I do trust God, for He is Lord! I do believe that the Lord heals, and that nothing is impossible with Him. One very good thing already took place that I can share. And this may help you: whatever the Lord has done for me, He can do for you.

It takes a lot more faith to go through surgery or trials and to believe and know that the Lord is with you, than to receive a healing. To face life-threatening surgery with the possibility of not making it, yet knowing that the Lord is with you, and then to experience the peace and confidence of God, is a miracle! Only the Lord can work that in you. We in ourselves are incapable of this.

James 1:2–4 talks about how, when we go through trials, we are to, "My brethren, count it all joy when you fall into various trials, knowing that the testing of your faith produces patience. But let patience have its perfect work, that you may be perfect and complete, lacking nothing" (NKJV).

James 1:12 says, "Blessed is a man who perseveres under trial: for once he has been approved, he will receive the crown of life, which the Lord has promised to those who love Him." Some interesting words here: "consider it all joy." Usually we do not consider trials a joy, but God says, "Consider it all joy." Jesus is our example, "Who for the joy that was set before Him endured the cross, despising the shame, and has sat down at the right hand of the throne of God" (Heb. 12:2, NKJV).

Why do you suppose He said that? Because He knew the outcome; He knew that He was in the perfect will of God. He knew why He was here.

Nehemiah, when reading the Word said, "So they read distinctly from the book, in the Law of God; and they gave the sense, and helped them to understand the reading. And Nehemiah, who was the governor, Ezra the priest and scribe, and the Levites who taught the people said to all the people, 'This day is holy to the LORD your God; do not mourn nor weep.' For all the people wept, when they heard the words of the Law. Then he said to them, 'Go your way, eat the fat, drink the sweet, and send portions to those for whom nothing is prepared; for this day is holy to our LORD. Do not sorrow, for the joy of the LORD is your strength'" (Neh. 8:8–10, NKJV).

They heard the Living Word that day! And they responded to the Lord. We can have that same confidence if we put our trust in the Lord, "For we walk by faith, not by sight" (2 Cor. 5:7, NKJV). And we keep on walking, trusting the Lord in everything, "that your joy may be made full" (John 15:11, NASB).

There is only one condition: stay in the Lord, and trust Him. Only then can we have this quiet confidence, knowing that all will be well. In Isaiah 26:3, it says, "You will keep him in perfect peace, whose mind is stayed on You, because he trusts in You" (NKJV). This is done by spending time in His Word, talking to God about everything, and then doing what He tells you to do. There is a safe place in God, "He who dwells in the secret place of the Most High, shall abide under the shadow of the Almighty" (Ps. 91:1, NKJV).

My prayer is that you might find that place in the Lord! Does that mean there will not be anymore problems? No, of course not. As long as we are in this fallen world there will be problems. The good news is that there is a place in the Lord where we can have peace no matter what is going on in our lives because the Lord will carry you through when you put your trust in Him.

And let us not get tired of doing what is right, for after a while we will reap a harvest of blessing if we don't get discouraged and give up.

–Galatians 6:9, TLB

So do not give up!

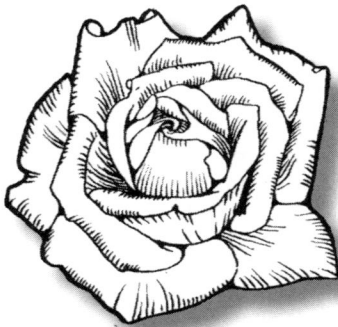

Chapter 10

Commitment

CANCER, OR FOR that matter any disease, affects the entire family. I saw this first hand as I grew up.

I was privileged to witness the commitment of my grandfather as he cared for his wife who was sick for years. It had a profound affect on me as a child.

My mother was visiting her sister and she had left us at the farm with our grandparents. We loved to go there and run on the farm and pick apples; it was a great place for us kids roaming around the farm, climbing trees.

Grandma always made breakfast for us, and so she did one morning, except she did something very strange. Instead of putting cheese on our bread, I noticed that she went to the soapbox by the sink, started slicing the soap and put it on the bread. Then she told us to eat it. My two brothers and I were very quiet and we could not believe our eyes.

She pushed the plates close to us with the soap sandwiches on it and she said eat it.

"You are kidding, right, Grandma?" I asked.

"No, you eat this," she said. Then I knew something was drastically wrong. I slipped from my chair and ran out to the field to my grandfather.

"You got to come, Grandpa. I think something's wrong with Grandmother. She put soap on our bread and she wants us to eat it."

Grandfather left his work immediately and followed me to the farmhouse. He saw that something was wrong right away and he called the doctor. Grandma was bedridden for several years thereafter. She was diagnosed with Alzheimer's. I was only twelve years old, and I observed a tremendous lesson in love and commitment of my grandfather as he took care of his wife. He never complained, was never angry or upset, and I noticed he read the Word of God a lot.

Many times, my grandfather would come in the house, pick up the Word of God, read a verse, and go back outside to attend the sheep. As I observed him, I knew that he was thinking about the Lord.

Grandmother did not recognize us anymore and would ask my mother, "Who are these children, and when are they going home?" My grandfather put the bed in the living room, so she could see everything that went on. We do not know how much she understood, but Grandfather ran the farm and took care of Grandma.

After about five years, a miracle happened. My grandmother totally recognized all her surroundings and she called her husband.

"Jan," she said. "I am going home today!" My grandfather pulled up a chair next to her bed and opened the

Bible and said, "Atje, let's read Psalm 116." This is what he read to her that day:

> I love the Lord because he hears my prayers and answers them. Because he bends down and listens, I will pray as long as I breathe! Death stared me in the face—I was frightened and sad. Then I cried, "Lord, save me!" How kind he is! How good he is! So merciful, this God of ours! The Lord protects the simple and the childlike; I was facing death, and then he saved me. Now I can relax. For the Lord has done this wonderful miracle for me. He has saved me from death, my eyes from tears, my feet from stumbling. I shall live! Yes, in his presence-here on earth! In my discouragement I thought, "They are lying when they say I will recover." But now what can I offer Jehovah for all he has done for me? I will bring him an offering of wine and praise his name for saving me. I will publicly bring him the sacrifice I vowed I would. His loved ones are very precious to him, and he does not lightly let them die. O Lord, you have freed me from my bonds, and I will serve you forever. I will worship you and offer you a sacrifice of thanksgiving. Here in the courts of the Temple in Jerusalem, before all the people, I will pay everything I vowed to the Lord. Praise the Lord.
>
> —PSALM 116, TLB

As he read this Psalm to my grandma, she was totally clear in her mind and recognized her husband. Total peace surrounded both of them. After he read these scriptures to her, he closed the Bible and both my grandfather and grandmother prayed together, they kissed each other good-bye, and she closed her eyes and peacefully went to be with Jesus!

I have never forgotten what took place that day. What a wonderful example of love and caring for your wife in the good days and in the not so good days. My grandmother had not recognized her husband or her children for over five years, until the end of her life, when God gave them a gift of knowing each other again and to be able to say good-bye, until they will see each other again in heaven.

When she passed on, my grandpa said, "We are not going to be upset, because grandma is with Jesus." Two months later my grandfather joined his wife.

In observing my grandfather's devotion for his wife and his faith in God, he was an example of what true commitment and love is. He did not preach, he did not say anything, but as a young girl I observed him and saw the love of God in action. Reading the Word, taking care of his wife, he never complained. I knew he loved the Lord. His example I will never forget. What a legacy he left behind.

The other man in my life is my husband. I am equally sure that my husband would do the same. When I was diagnosed with breast cancer he was there to pray for me, listen to me, and support me, no matter what decision I would make.

Husbands can be a great help to their wives, to assist them in making the right choices; not based on looks, but based on what is best for their health in facts, and not on feelings. They can be a great support in letting their wife know, "I love you, honey, no matter what!"

Just listen to your wife, let her talk, and take time with her as both of you go through a very difficult time of making decisions. Women need to talk to process things.

The day I came home after brain surgery my husband was more elated than I was. He kept on saying: "I am so glad you are home and that you are OK! I thank the Lord! Thank You, God!"

I watched him and saw the toll that it had also taken on him. He was so relieved that I was fine. Not once, but over and over again, he thanked the Lord and hugged me, and hugged me.

Sometimes, when women go through breast cancer, or whatever it may be, we can be so busy with ourselves that we forget all about the people around us: our husbands, our children, our parents. We can make things easy for them also, by letting them talk and to pray with them and talk as a family and bring it all to the Lord. The whole family is involved. It will allow the Lord to work His way and His will out in all of our lives.

The man who finds life will find
it through trusting God.

—Romans 1:17, TLB

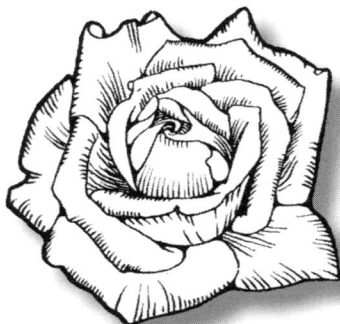

Chapter 11

I Will Trust God

IT WAS SIX o'clock and we had just finished dinner. There were candles on the table, which I love. All of a sudden, Simen announced, "How would you like to go out to see a movie?" We had not gone to see a movie for I don't know how long. It sounded like a great idea, so we decided on a movie at the mall in Orange, and coffee afterwards.

It was a brisk, cold December evening in California. As we walked to the movie theater, engaged in an amicable conversation, I suddenly fell to the ground and lost consciousness for a second. People came running up to us, and asked if we needed an ambulance. My husband tried to get me off the ground, but that was the wrong thing to do. I felt like taking it easy; I needed a little time to adjust. When I opened my eyes, I saw all these people looking at me. One man said, "Let me call 9-1-1 for you."

"No," I said. "I'll be fine, but thank you." After I sat down on a bench, still shaky from the ordeal, we decided to go home. That was our evening out.

"I'll call the doctor first thing in the morning," my husband said. This was not the first time this had happened. I had talked to a doctor before about this, and they were never able to find the problem, but I decided to give it another try.

I made an appointment for the next week. As the doctor looked over my chart, he said, "Has this happened before?"

"Yes, about a year ago," I said. "I was going for a walk in our neighborhood when I fell. Trying to catch my breath, I sat down in the street. When I got up too fast, the wind was knocked out of my lungs. Since I did not black out totally, I did not think about it too much." After the doctor listened to me, he said, "I will send you to a cardiologist. I think it is your heart." My heart checked out fine, so I left it alone and forgot about it.

Then one day, as I walked up to our home with my two little grandsons by my side, I fell again. The two little boys called to my daughter, "Mom, please come! Hurry! Oma fell down! Hurry!"

Again I made an appointment to see our doctor. This time I insisted that I wanted to find out why I had these blackouts. There had to be a reason for all of this.

"I will send you to a neurologist. Maybe he can help you," my doctor said, and he handed me a piece of paper with the doctor's name and phone number. "Give him a call. He might be able to help you."

The next day I made the appointment with a neurologist.

"We can see you next Thursday," the receptionist said. "Will ten thirty be all right?"

"Yes," I said. "I will see you then." The doctor was a nice man who took time to listen, did the usual tests in the office, and said, "Mrs. De Vries, I do not think we will find anything wrong with you, but I suggest we take an MRI of your brain. But again, I do not think we will find anything wrong with you. You appear to be in good health." He gave me a hand, and I left. The girl in the front office made the appointment for me.

"Is next Wednesday OK?" she asked, as I was about to leave.

"That's fine," I said.

I had never had an MRI as far as I knew, and did not know what they were going to do. In fact I did not give it much thought.

My test was scheduled for early the following week. As I arrived at the hospital and was ushered into this room, all I saw was what looked to me like a huge machine.

"You want me to go in there?" I asked the radiologist.

She looked at me with a smile. "It's only one hour and maybe another twenty minutes, and you'll be done."

I climbed up on the table, and she put a towel over my head, locked my head in this little cage, and clamped it shut.

"Don't move," she said. "Lay very still. If you need anything, push this knob." With that she handed me this tiny push button, and off she went, leaving me inside this huge machine. I prayed and prayed the whole time I was in there. After about an hour, which to me felt like hours, I heard them say, "One more, minute, Mrs. De Vries, and you will be ready to go." I must say, I could not wait to get out of that machine. It was huge! I felt trapped in there and was glad to be out of it.

I hurried home and resumed what I was doing that day, which was painting our living room. Soon the phone rang again.

"Mrs. De Vries, this is radiology. Can you come in tomorrow morning for an MRI?"

"An MRI?" I asked. "I was just in for an MRI."

There was a pause on the other end of the line. "The MRI revealed what looked like a lesion on the front lobe of your brain, and your doctor wants to take some more pictures. And Mrs. De Vries, this time it will only be twenty minutes. Is nine o'clock all right for you?"

"Sure," I said. As I got off the phone, my husband, who had heard the phone conversation, said, "You have to do it over?"

"Yeah, they found a lesion on my brain...or did she say two lesions? Maybe it was a mistake. Who knows? We don't know what is going on, so let's wait until tomorrow."

What about this brain lesion? Once you have had breast cancer, any tumor is suspicious. I knew that. Could there be a connection? We prayed together, Simen and I, and brought it before the Lord to seek His wisdom, for us and the doctor. Our daughter, Jacqueline, walked into the living room and overheard part of our conversation.

"What was that all about?" she asked. "Didn't you already have an MRI?"

"Yes, I did, but they want some more pictures tomorrow." There was no need to worry her. She was visiting us that week and was going to meet some friends that evening. We did not feel like spoiling her evening, because we didn't know if there was anything to be concerned about. The next morning we arrived at the hospital for some additional tests. That afternoon, after the test, we hoped and prayed for a good result. Then the phone rang! *Oh,* I thought, *not a good sign, especially if the doctor is on the other end of the line for they never call unless it is serious.*

"Mrs. De Vries?" the voice said, "this is your doctor. We indeed discovered two nodules at the frontal lobes of your brain. Can you come to my office tomorrow? I want to go over some of the tests I want you to have." As I hung up the phone, I thought, *This is so unreal, not one but two nodules! I feel fine, so it cannot be that serious.* It still amazes me that when you least expect it, this happens. I had no idea what was going on. Yes, there were some puzzling incidents that had happened recently, but maybe this was the reason. Or was there another reason for it, as the doctor later suggested? Whatever the case, it was good that we found the two nodules in my brain, because they can cause a great deal of trouble, as I found out. My doctor suggested that I see a brain surgeon in the Fullerton area. The girl in the front office gave me the phone number and my MRI.

Coming home, I immediately made an appointment to see the surgeon.

"I have an opening tomorrow morning, like eight o'clock," the receptionist said. "Can you make it?"

"Sure, we'll be there," I said.

I love to read and enjoy a cup of coffee in the morning. I take my Bible and my favorite book of-the-moment, and enjoy myself. It is a routine that I have had for years. I love the early mornings. I also love to read. Our living room is full of books.

That morning was no different. As I was about to see the brain surgeon, I read a story about Helen Keller, the lady who was born blind and deaf. It is the remarkable story of a young girl, and what she did with her handicap. She founded The Braille Institute, for people who are blind.[1]

As I was reading that story, I thanked the Lord for my eyesight. It must be terrible to lose your sight; it is something you really never think about. I closed my eyes. Could I handle losing my sight? What a remarkable young woman Helen Keller must have been! What are we doing with our so-called handicaps in this life? Are we using them for the good?

At eight o'clock, we arrived at the brain surgeon's office. I am sure they squeezed me in early, as I saw no one else there that early. Up to that moment, I did not really understand where the tumors were located. The doctor told me they were right at the optic nerve.

"What does this involve?" I asked him.

"It means," the doctor explained, "that it could interfere with your eye sight."

"My eyes," I asked?

"Yes," he explained. "The tumors are right between the optic nerve and the carotid arteries. Not a good place, because if it fastened itself on the optic nerve and if we cannot get it all, the possibility is that it will grow back. It is very rare indeed that you have two tumors instead of one, on either side." He continued, "I would suggest you see an ophthalmologist to have your eyes checked and have a vision field test done."

"What can you find out from that?" I asked.

"We can see how much the optic nerve is involved. Call me when you have this done and I will see you in about one week," he said.

I made an appointment with the eye specialist. I had an eye examination and a visual field test. This test indicated that the tumors were against the optic nerves, but how close we did not know.

In the meantime, Simen and I decided to do some research on our own, going to the bookstore and reading medical books. We found a book on neurosurgery, and in it were some of the best doctors in their field. One of them was a Doctor Steven Giannotta. We made a notation of it just in case we needed a good doctor, and then headed home.

A week later, we again met with the brain surgeon, who by now had collected my file. The surgeon looked over all my medical reports and I could see he was having a difficult time with it.

"Where exactly, doctor, are those tumors?" I asked.

"At a very difficult spot," he said. "They are extra-axial, markedly enhancing masses posterior to the anterior clinoid bilaterally. The left mass is larger than the right. These may represent meningiomas or neurofibromas. Metastic disease is not excluded."

"What if I do not have the surgery?" I questioned the doctor.

"There is a possibility that you could lose your sight."

"Can you do the surgery?" I asked.

He scratched his head but did not say anything for a moment. "I do not want to lose you on the operating table," was his response.

"Did you ever do this kind of brain surgery before?" I asked.

"Yes, of course. I make a living doing brain surgery," he said. He looked at me and said, "But it is a very difficult surgery."

He then got his computer out and looked up something. It took a while before he looked up at me and said, "There is a doctor, named Dr. Giannotta, at the USC Medical Center in Los Angeles, who is the foremost authority in brain surgery of this kind. I can give you a referral to see him. I do not know if you can go there because, as I understand it, you have an HMO."

When you are in a HMO, you cannot go to any doctor of your choice. As he handed me the name of the doctor, we knew it was the same doctor we had looked up in the bookstore the week before. We took his advice, thanked him for the referral and his help, and left. Coming home we called the insurance company just to be sure. We explained our plight, and they said yes, we would be able to visit the doctor of our choice.

The next thing I did was make an appointment with Dr. Giannotta at the USC Medical Center. The girl on the phone was very friendly and said, "We have an opening tomorrow morning. Can you make it? Bring with you all of your MRIs, vision field test, and so on."

I went to the hospital where the MRI was taken and asked if I could take it to USC Medical Center with the medical report. "Sure, we can have it ready for you this afternoon at two o'clock." As I picked up my report I was able to read the MRI, and it said, "Possible a meningioma or a fibro adenoma, but we cannot rule out metastasis."

The fact that I had breast cancer a couple of year's prior means the possibility of a recurrence of cancer is always a possibility. I have never entertained that thought, but looking back now, I know this was the Lord. I was so sure it was not cancer, and I just had this assurance that I was going to be all right!

As we approached USC Medical Center, I thought, *What is the doctor going to say?* As we walked into his office I felt at home, and when I met Dr. Giannotta, I instantly liked him. He was a man of few words and very confident in what he was doing. I trusted him immediately! I thought, *If any one can do this, he can.*

After going over my medical history, he looked at me and said, "Next Monday?"

I gasped. "Next Monday?" I asked. "You mean, this Monday?"

"The earlier, the better," was his reply. "We will remove one tumor at a time. We will first remove the left tumor because that is the largest one, and when you recuperate after a year we might remove the right one."

"Can we do them at the same time?" I asked.

"No, we have to wait and do two surgeries."

This took me by surprise. "I have things to do," I said. "I'm a bookkeeper, and this will take a lot of time to recuperate. How about in four weeks?" I asked.

"Don't wait too long," he said. "It is better earlier than later, if you are going to do it. The receptionist will schedule you for surgery." We shook hands and left the room.

I was somewhat taken back by how fast the doctor wanted to proceed with the surgery, and yet I was impressed with his confident attitude. I did not detect any hesitance in his voice, which gave me confidence to go ahead with the surgery.

My husband decided to get some lunch, during which we talked at great length about the upcoming surgery. I had so many questions, and I had so much to do. I do the bookkeeping for our company, and we produce a one-hour weekly Christian television program for Amsterdam and the surrounding cities, along with a weekly half-hour program for TBN Europe. I wondered, *After this surgery, will I still be able to do all these things? Will I be able to resume my life as before the surgery?*

A week earlier, our company had a tax audit, which we were not able to finish, so the auditor said, "I will come back in two weeks and finish it."

"In two weeks," I replied, "I probably will have my brain surgery."

"Oh, you will be fine," he said, "I will call you." There were so many plans to be made, but finally I had to give it all over to God. I like things orderly, nicely lined up, but life can throw you for a loop and that is what happened to me this time. So many unanswered questions—I had to "let go and let God."

That same evening, our daughter Jacqueline called. "Mom, you are still coming, right?" We had two tickets to fly to Iowa, where she lived. I shared with her what the doctor had said that morning, "I don't know if I can come, honey, maybe I should postpone the trip til after surgery," I said.

"But Mom, I have organized a prayer meeting for you and all the women will come and pray for you; you just have to come."

I thought for a minute, it would be nice to see my daughter again and I sure need prayer, so I said, "OK, I'll be there." I postponed the surgery a couple of weeks and my husband and I flew out the following week to Cedar Rapids.

The women come together every week to study the Bible and pray, so when they heard that I needed surgery, they all came and prayed over me, and for all the doctors involved; what a blessing! And I knew that I was going to be fine, I did not know how the Lord was going to work this out, but of one thing I was certain—God is in control. Looking around the room, seeing all these women praying for me, and my daughter Jacqueline, I felt so blessed. How could I go wrong? What a privilege to go to God in prayer!

The following morning, I opened the Word to Ephesians 1, where it says that Paul prayed for the church in Ephesus, "That the God of our Lord Jesus Christ, the Father of glory, may give to you the spirit of wisdom and revelation in the knowledge of Him, the eyes of your understanding being enlightened; that you may know what is the hope of His calling, what are the riches of the glory of His inheritance in the saints, and what is the exceeding greatness of His power toward us who believe, according to the working of His mighty power" (Eph. 1:17–19, NKJV).

The apostle Paul expresses here that we can know Christ and understand His purpose and power in our life. Such revelation will produce insight in what the Lord tells us to do.

The eyes of your heart, referring to the inner man, can know what the plan is, that God has for our life. That is why we are admonished, "Do not be conformed to this world, but be transformed by the renewing of your mind, that you may prove what is that good and acceptable and perfect will of God" (Rom. 12:2, NKJV). That inner you, when transformed by the power of God, "Christ in you, the hope of glory" (Col. 1:27, NKJV).

So you can know the will of God in a certain situation for "Your eyes saw my unformed substance, and in Your book all the days were written before ever they took shape, when as yet there was none of them" (Ps. 139:16).

I remember a missionary, years ago who was diagnosed with a brain tumor. After much prayer and fasting, the Lord said to him, *Go ahead and go to the mission field, and as you go, I will heal you.* He obeyed, and God healed him.

God spoke and it was done. For example, in Genesis 1 it states that God created the heavens and the earth. He first moved by His Spirit and then He spoke the Word and all things came into being. (See Genesis 1:2–3.) The Spirit still moves first, followed by God's Word. And God still moves by the same principles today.

"By faith" means trusting God. The Lord says in Isaiah 55:3, "Hear and your soul shall live" The psalmist also exhorts the people to faith saying, "Today, if you will hear His voice" (Ps. 95:7, NKJV).

There are many illustrations of faith in the Bible and if we study the life of Abraham we can see how it grows in the life of a believer. What did God teach him? "Now it was not written for his sake alone that it was imputed to him, but also for us. It shall be imputed to us who believe in Him who raised up Jesus our Lord from the dead" (Rom. 4:23–24, NKJV).

Abraham is called the friend of God. God made known His will to Abraham over and over again. (See James 2:23.) What made this man so pleasing to God? Just this, he believed God; what He says, He will do it! We also receive from God in the same way. "Or has He spoken and shall He not make it good?" (Num. 23:19).

When God called Abraham unto Himself and promised him a land that God Himself would show him, the Scripture says, Abraham departed as the Lord had spoken to him. And just as God called Abraham; He calls us. It is not written only for him, but to all who God calls.

The stories of the Old Testament are written for us as an example.

All of us are destined for a purpose. God alone knows the future. When we, like Abraham, give our lives over to God, Who knows us best, then we're a blessed people. "Seek ye the kingdom of God" (Luke 12:31, KJV).

Abraham went, as God called him, to a place he did not know. He was most likely approached by friends and neighbors who asked him where he was going. Abraham must have answered, "I don't know, but we are going to a land that God will show us." Each one of us has a call to follow the Lord; only those who obey the Lord, will find a sense of destiny, a purpose and a plan. But before I go any further, I want to explain something about faith and presumption.

So many people seem to be somewhat surprised by the fact that God still speaks today! Why pray or talk to God, if we don't believe that He hears and talks to us. Somehow we have the idea that God is so far removed from us that He cannot possibly be interested in you or me, but Yes, He is! The Psalmist says, "What is man that You are mindful of him, and the son of man that You visit him?" (Ps. 8:4, NKJV). Because of this, some substitute presumption for faith. The words already explain what I am trying to say—Faith is to believe God. For what does Scripture say? "Abraham believed God and it was accounted to him for righteousness" (Rom. 4:3, KJV).

When the apostle Paul was taken as a prisoner to Rome with some other prisoners, he warned them not to go a certain way because he perceived that this voyage will end in disaster, but the men would not listen to him. And when the storm came, Paul said that they should have listened to him, and not sailed from Crete and incurred their disaster and loss. But he said, "I have good news for you, For there stood by me this night an angel of the God to whom I belong and whom I serve. Saying, "Do not be afraid, Paul; you must be brought before Caesar; and indeed God has granted you all those who sail with you. Therefore take heart, men, for I believe God that it will be just as it was told me" (Acts 27:24–25, NKJV). Paul received a word from God that all would be well.

Presumption is when we suppose, guess, or presume what God has spoken. How then? You may say, "Well, when we go to the Word—God's Word—we can pick a verse that we like, and then we can quote it over and over again, because it is what we want." But, the question is: Did God give you this verse? The word *logos* means the Word of God, and the word *rhema* refers to the living Word when spoken to us, as it was in Abraham's case.

The Lord appeared to Abraham in a dream and said, "You will be the father of many nations" (Gen. 12:2). Abraham did not produce this or conjure this up. No, God spoke to him, and that is called a living word (rhema). We can have a living relationship with God like Abraham.

Years ago, I needed a word and healing for our son when he was diagnosed with scleroderma. Many people prayed for me and for our son saying, "Believe God he is healed!" Yet the words that came to me from God's Word was, "not my will, but Yours, be done" (Luke 22:42, NKJV). Over and over again this verse went through my mind. It was not until I relinquished our son to God, that the Lord began to heal him without surgery or medicine, but I did have to give him over to God.

I did not have a Word, yet I trusted God. Here is where faith comes in. I trusted God, no matter what He decided was for our good. Total peace engulfed me—it was a miracle. Whether God would heal our son or take him home to be with Jesus, I knew it was in God's hands, so I totally trusted the Lord. I could not have done this on my own; God did a miracle in my heart. After three months, God spoke to me and said, *I am going to heal him.* In surrendering our son to God, He healed him. What a miracle!

Faith, then, is not having it our way, but seeking God's way in what He wants us to do, and then waiting for His answer.

I had a whole series of tests, to identify if I was truly ready and able to trust the Lord for my brain surgery: Am I willing to go through the surgery? Do I still trust the Lord? Do I experience the peace of God in my life? Am I able to surrender my life to the Lord, when all does not go the way I would like it to go? Do I still praise the Lord?

My unwillingness in not going to the doctor could also have meant that I was afraid. I could have hid behind the phrase, "I trust the Lord and I am not going to a doctor." And yet people have been healed, set free who do not even know much about God. God will meet you wherever you are in life, for He is a merciful God.

100

In my difficult journey of brain surgery, I was confident in the Lord. Weeks before the surgery I had a dream, and in my dream I saw a man and a woman walking up a hill. As I looked a little closer I recognized myself in the dream. I looked up into the man's face and I knew He was a different man. He was perfect. It was as if I could see right through Him. There was no sin in Him for He was the Lord. The girl was dark, a sinner, and I recognized it was me.

In my dream the Lord guided me up this steep hill, undergirding me until we arrived at the top. He took a step to the side and looked at me with His kind eyes.

I knew God was with me, and I was not alone. When I looked at Him and our eyes met, He smiled. It was as if He said, *You can make it, I will be with you.*

When I awoke the next morning, I knew I was not alone. The Lord was with me. He knew all about it and He was not surprised. The Lord is in control of our lives, even when we do not understand it; in fact we don't need to understand, all we need to do is *trust the Lord!*

Out of your innermost being can come a gift from God. It has nothing to do with the human mind, nor the power of reason, but a knowing that God is in control! In the Book of Lamentations there was a person named Jeremiah. The whole world collapsed around him. He reached deep inside of himself, and a surprising revelation took place in his spirit, "yet there is one ray of hope; His compassion never ends. It is only the Lord's mercies that have kept us from complete destruction. Great is His faithfulness; His loving kindness begins afresh each day.

The Lord is wonderfully good to those who wait for Him, to those who seek for Him" (Lam. 3:21–25, TLB). This is the passage from which this beloved hymn comes from:

> Great is Thy faithfulness,
> Great is Thy faithfulness.
> Morning by morning new mercies I see.
> All I have needed Thy hand has provided,
> Great is Thy faithfulness Lord unto me.[2]

For we walk by faith, not by sight.

—2 Corinthians 5:7, NKJV

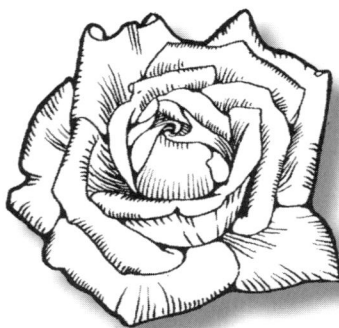

Chapter 12

Brain Surgery

IT WAS MAY 18, 2001, the day of the surgery arrived. Our daughter, Yvonne, and son, Simon, came the evening before. We prayed and we talked until late in the evening. The rest of the family came to the hospital the next morning. It was difficult for our children, as they needed assurance and support. Yet, it was a great opportunity to minister to them and to point them to the Lord. I was able to pray with them and to assure them that all would be well. I did not know how long the recuperation was going to take, but I reminded our children of this surety that no matter what, God is good!

Surgery was at ten o'clock that morning. After they prepared me for surgery, the anesthesiologist came by and said, "We are about to wheel her into surgery. You want to say a prayer now?" We all joined hands, asking the Lord to bless the surgeons and the nurses, to guide them and give them wisdom. We asked God to grant me a speedy recovery, and then off we went. The last thing I remember was what the anesthesiologist said to the nurses: "This is a very clean lady. She does not smoke or drink, but now

I will give her a cocktail." He meant a combination of drugs for the anesthesia. Some hours later, in the recovery room, I heard them telling me to move my toes, fingers, and eyes. They wanted to see if everything was working.

As my husband and family were escorted to the lobby of the hospital to wait until the surgery was over, they handed my husband a small pager. "When this goes off, it will let you know that the surgery is over and the doctor is on his way to talk to you" the nurse at the front desk explained. Everyone watched that pager. After about three hours, the pager went off and the doctor was on the way.

The door of the elevator opened, and Dr. Giannotta came out with a smile. "Everything went well," he said," and she is responding just fine."

I was hospitalized five days. The first time I looked in the mirror I was surprised, thinking all my hair would be gone, but they only shaved half my head. One family member remarked, "You have a perfectly round head."

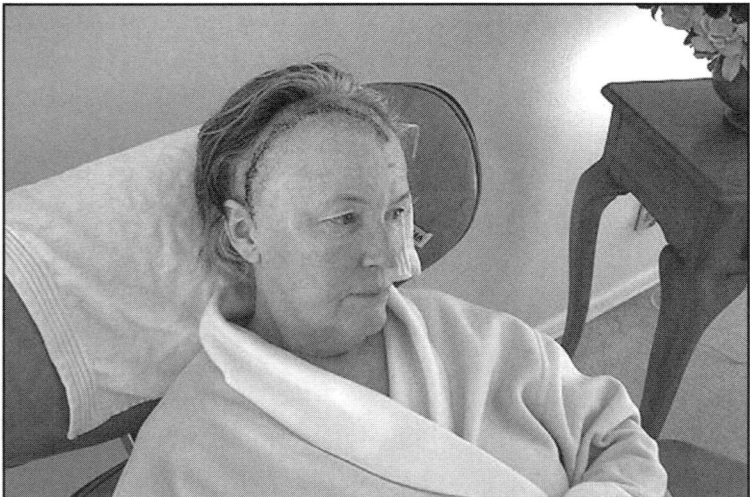

We also sent a thank you note to all the doctors who had helped me. In the recovery room, one of the nurses came in and said, "Mrs. De Vries, I prayed for you during the surgery." She assisted the doctor in the surgery room. I was touched by so many kind and helpful people. The next day the doctor came with his assistant.

"How are you doing, Mrs. De Vries?"

"Fine," I said, wanting to know more of how he felt the surgery went.

"All went fine," he explained, "and the tumor was a meningioma."

"May I have the pathology report?"

"Sure," he said. "It will take a few days, and I will make sure you will get one."

When I received the pathology report it said the tumor had completely covered the optic nerve and carotid artery as well as the third nerve. The optic nerve was completely decompressed, and the anterior clinoid itself was drilled away. As I was reading the report, I thanked the Lord for helping me. I felt very fortunate to have had the surgery and to have a good doctor and God to help us. The next day I was up and walking about. It was a speedy recovery.

When I came home, our daughter prepared a good dinner for us. I needed vitamins, she told me, to recuperate. We all thanked the Lord for a successful surgery. My husband was so happy, thanking the Lord throughout the day. After being home a couple of days, my daughter Jacqueline decided it was time for me to have a haircut. My hair was long on one side, short on the other side, and where they did surgery, it was totally shaved off. From the middle of my head to the side down below my ear, there was no hair. Now, remember, I was still groggy from the anesthesia and pain medication. I did not really care how I looked.

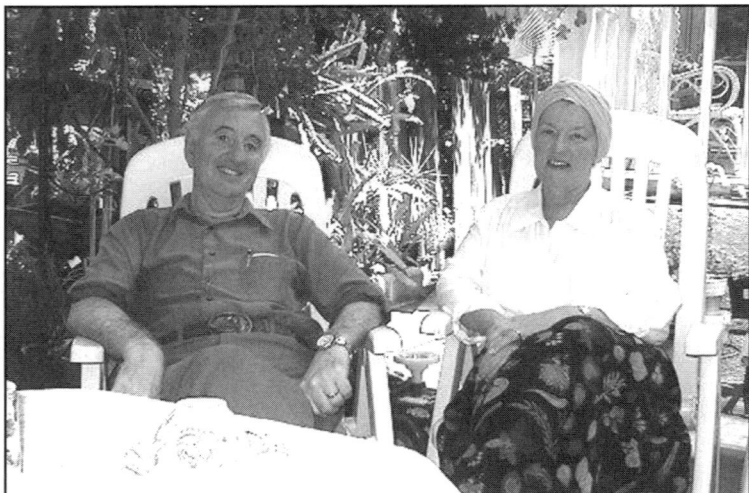

"I am not going to a hair dresser," I commented. "If you think I need a haircut, you do it!"

She looked at me with big eyes. "Me? You want me to cut your hair?"

"Well, it's like this," I said. "You cut my hair or we leave it the way it is, because I am not going to a hair dresser. Besides, my stitches are still in my head until next week, and the wound is very tender."

Jacqueline got the scissors and said, "All right, I'll cut your hair." After I got a towel around my shoulders, she began cutting my hair. I noticed there seemed to be no stopping her, so I finally said, "Maybe you better stop now because it feels like I will have no hair left."

"I'm sorry, Mom," she said. "I think I cut too much hair. You want to see? Let me get you a mirror." She disappeared, letting me sit there. *I should not have had her cut my hair,* I thought to myself.

"Here, Mom," she said, and handed me a mirror. "I am sorry, mom," she said. "I did cut too much, huh?"

"It's okay, Jacqueline," I said. "You tried." I looked in the mirror at my almost bald head and thought, *I can put a scarf over my head.* I really did not care, probably because of the medication in my system. When my family saw me they said, "Mom, who cut your hair?"

"I did," Jacqueline said, and we all laughed!

"I can always buy a wig," I said. "No problem."

The only experience I ever had with a wig was several years ago when we had a guest staying with us for a week. We did not know him that well, but a friend introduced him to us and asked if he could stay at our home for a week. We said yes, and looked forward to his coming. It was the week before Christmas, and he was going to spend the holidays with us. He lives in Holland, and since we also are Dutch, it is nice to have someone over from the place we were born. We had a nice time, but I noticed that our new friend had a difficult time relaxing. It was as if he tried to portray a certain image; it was difficult for him to be himself, I noticed. He was always dressed immaculately, with a suit and tie, every day.

On Christmas Eve, I was preparing dinner when our friend walked into the kitchen.

"Is there enough time for me to take a shower?" he asked.

"Sure," I said. "Dinner is not until six o'clock."

Six o'clock came. Then six fifteen, and we became worried. Not only was dinner ready, but our friend did not come out of the bathroom. We all sat around the dinner table wondering what could possibly have happened to him.

"Maybe you should check on him," I said to my husband. Then the door opened and our guest appeared. We all burst out laughing, including our guest, as he had no hair. He looked so different, and in his hand he had a dark wig. One of our family members commented, "That looks like a dead rat," to which my husband replied, "You boys be nice!"

"What happened?" we asked.

"I washed my wig," he said, "and sprayed it with hairspray. The wig shrunk, and I tried to dry it, but it was no use."

We could only imagine what he went through in that bathroom, wondering what we would think when he came out without his wig. We all had a good laugh, and the ice was broken between all of us. We had a marvelous Christmas Eve, and I might add, our friend now felt right at home with us, so it all turned out for the good.

In the future I would have another brain surgery. They performed the first surgery on the left side of my brain, and the right side was still in question. We could only hope that it was a slow growing tumor. Every six

months, I needed an MRI of my brain to check the prog-
ress, keeping an eye on the other tumor. But for the
time being, I was doing great. All I did was recuperate,
thanking the Lord for healing me with no complications
at all. Even my headaches disappeared after about four
weeks, and I might add that I am doing exceptionally
well.

Finally, my brethren,
be strong in the Lord and in
the power of His might.

–Ephesians 6:10, NKJV

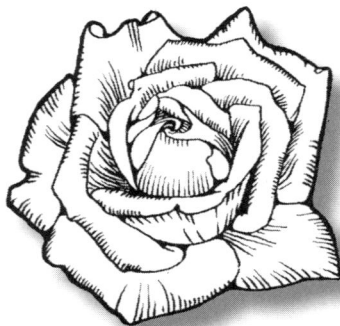

Chapter 13

God Is My Strength

"WELL, MRS. DE VRIES, are you ready for your next surgery?" It was almost two years since I had my first brain surgery. Dr. Giannotta, looked at me, and I was taken a little bit aback. Yes, I made a chart of my progress, and kept a diagram of the size of the other tumor, which seemed to grow slightly. I felt fine, so it was a good time to proceed if I decided to have it done. There was always the danger that the tumor would fasten itself to the optic nerve or carotid artery, with the result that the surgeon is not able to get all of the tumor. Then there would be a chance that the tumor could grow back faster. The size of the tumor is not as important as where the tumor is located. Some tumors grow to considerable size, yet do not cause problems, while others are small but troublesome because they are in a difficult place, as mine was.

I arrived at the hospital with my husband and son. Our other children, and my brother and sister, came right behind us. Also, our pastors, Bob Barnett and Kenny

Wilson, came and prayed for me, so I had a great support system.

The nurse came in to draw blood. The anesthesiologist came and asked several questions. Another nurse came and explained all the complications of the surgery.

"You know, Mrs. De Vries, there always is a small chance of you not coming out alive, or having a stroke."

"Yes, I know," I said. I was very aware of the complications that could transpire. My daughter was sitting next to my bed crying. I told her, "Do not worry, Yvonne, I will be fine, really." I was confident that the Lord was in control.

The day before I was going into surgery, I was reading Habakkuk 3:17–19 (NKJV). I was really touched by the scripture that explained what I felt that day. Handing the Bible over to one of the pastors, I said, "Kenny, can you read this for me?" As he began to read, I still felt the same way:

> Though the fig tree may not blossom, Nor fruit be on the vines; Though the labor of the olive may fail, And the fields yield no food; Though the flock may be cut off from the fold, And there be no herd in the stalls—Yet will I rejoice in the LORD, I will joy in the God of my salvation. The LORD God is my strength; He will make my feet like deer's feet, And He will make me walk on my high hills.

One of the doctors came to get me, but before he did he asked, "Do you all want to say a prayer before I take her?"

"Yes," they responded, and they all prayed for me, and for the doctors and nurses. Hours later I woke up in the intensive care unit. I was nauseated but had no pain. They kept me sedated, asking me questions: Who is the president? Where are you? They were checking to see if I still was thinking. I dozed in and out of consciousness.

The surgery went extremely well. This tumor also was a meningioma, and the tumor was completely removed. Thank You, Jesus!

As I woke up the next morning, I looked over at the bed next to me. I saw a young mother who, like me, just came out of brain surgery. As we started to talk she said, "I am so afraid," Over and over again she kept saying, "I am so scared! I am so scared!" As she shared with me, I found out that she was a born-again believer, yet fear had a grip on her life.

She listened intently as I shared with her what the Word of God has to say about fear, that fear is a spirit, and that, "God has not given us a spirit of fear, but of power and of love and of a sound mind " (2 Tim. 1:7, NKJV). I then asked her if I could pray for her, and she said yes. We both prayed that God would set her free.

When you are weak in body and soul because of illness, or surgery, Satan will take advantage of it. When you dwell on a negative report instead of trusting God, and filling your mind on things of this world, you open a door through which fear can sneak in. That is way it is so important to share your fears with someone, and bring it to God in prayer. Half the battle is won when you expose Satan.

Fear is something you cannot see. You are dealing with something intangible, it is a spirit. Many times we fear things that will never take place.

But how then, do we deal with fear? First, we have to understand that our weapons are not physical but spiritual.

Whenever the devil sees an opening in your life, he moves in playing havoc with your thought life, if you let him. Therefore God says, "Do not be conformed to this world, but be transformed by the renewing of your mind" (Rom. 12:2, NKJV). We deal with fear by submitting to God first. It is by His strength that we overcome Satan, not in our strength. We are admonished to resist the devil, and to take a stand and start praising the Lord. The devil will suggest anything he can, to distract you. He will do all he can to bombard your mind with negative thoughts.

The battle is in your thought life, you are the only one that can take it captive and resist it, think on the good things in life immediately, and do not entertain negative thoughts or let your mind wander in all directions.

You have a choice, it does not mean that you do not face reality, but with God all things are possible! God has the final say over our circumstances. Too many people love to dwell on the negative things in their life and entertain it. You do not have to, you can resist it and draw a line in the sand saying, Enough is enough! In Jesus name!

Then you put up your hands and start praising the Lord. Psalm 103 says, "Bless the Lord, O my soul: and all that is within me, bless his holy name" (KJV). Satan has to go. It is not maybe—he will! Because one thing he does not like is praising God.

How then do we take our thought life captive? First of all, by subjecting yourself to God, reading the Word of God, "Thy word is a lamp unto my feet, and a light unto my path" (Ps. 119:105, KJV).

As I was talking to this young mom, I was reminded again of a similar situation some years ago when our daughter came home one day from work saying, "Dad, can you lead my boss to the Lord? She does not know God."

"You think she will?" Dad asked her.

"Yes, I am sure," she said. Simen went to see the lady, and sure enough, after she heard the gospel, she accepted the Lord and was born again.

It was some time later that she was diagnosed with cancer. Fear began to grip her and she was afraid of driving, which was very unusual for her, because her job required a lot of traveling. Our daughter again told us about the predicament she was in.

We visited her in the hospital, and as she began to share with us she started to cry. "I couldn't tell any one this," she said, "because people might think I am crazy, and I am not. I am so fearful! And I cannot drive my car anymore!" We let her talk about all the fears she had, and then I asked her a question, "Do you believe that this is the devil?"

She stopped crying and looked at me and said, "Yes, I know he is tormenting me, and I was not able to share this with anyone until today."

I shared with her that "We do not wrestle against flesh and blood, but against principalities, against powers, against the rulers of the darkness of this age, against spiritual hosts of wickedness in the heavenly places" (Eph. 6:12, NKJV). As we submit ourselves to the Lord, and resist the devil, he will flee from us. "Can I pray for you?" I asked.

"Sure," she said. She was ready for prayer. We rebuked the devil and asked the Lord to set her free in Jesus' name, and the Lord set her free.

Later we heard that she was driving again and doing everything she used to do.

When you are living in fear, Satan has you bound. Fear is a spirit, and unless you realize this and face it head on, it will destroy your peace. Stand still for a moment, look at it see where it comes from and who is behind it. Once you expose the enemy, once he knows you know, he will leave you alone. We have to resist and take a stand. Do not forget to first submit yourself to God, for then the enemy has to flee!

We have a choice: we either yield to God or to the devil. We can yield to the Lord or we can give in to fear. If we open the door to the enemy, fear will move in. Therefore, as Philippians 4:8 says, "Finally, brethren, whatever things are true, whatever things are noble, whatever things are just, whatever things are pure, whatever things are lovely, whatever things are of good report, if there is any virtue and if there is anything praiseworthy— meditate on these things."

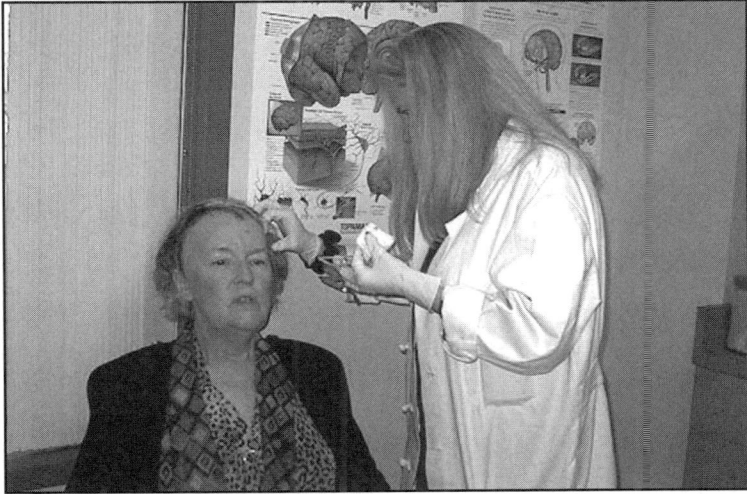

Ten days later the stitches were removed. I was about to leave when the Physician Assistant, Dawn Fishback, asked me to wait for the doctor. After a few minutes, Dr. Giannotta opened the door and said, "Wow, brain surgery didn't do you any harm!"

It was a great success. I felt great, and except for the scarf around my head, no one ever suspected that I just came out of brain surgery! I thanked Dr. Giannotta for all he had done. He was greatly used by God to perform this delicate brain surgery.

For about four weeks I experienced terrific headaches, but this I knew would be the result of the surgery and would pass. Prior to the first surgery, I asked the Physician Assistant, Dawn Fishback, if there would be any pain after brain surgery.

"Of course," she said, "you are going to have brain surgery, so you will have headaches." Then she added, "That will be a good sign."

"All right," I said, "I have headaches now, so what else is new?"

The headaches were especially severe at night. I slept for a couple of hours, and I would wake up with a bad headache, take some pain medication and fell back to sleep. That was the only problem I had. I would like to end this book with a great promise from God:

> For I know the thoughts that I think toward you, says the LORD, thoughts of peace and not of evil, to give you a future and a hope.
> —Jeremiah 29:11, NKJV

Afterword

DO I HAVE a guarantee that the cancer will never come back, or that no other nodules will appear? No, life is uncertain. But one thing is certain—God. He is always there for you, and He will help you.

At the moment of this writing, it has been eleven years that I have been cancer free! I feel good, never worried about cancer or even afraid of it, because my life is in God's hands. Doctors can only perform a diagnosis and do the surgery, but the Lord is the Healer.

My prayer is that in sharing my story of breast cancer with you, it will help you to look to the Lord. Nothing is impossible with God, for He is the great Physician! If you discover a nodule, do not wait six months for a confirmation. Have it checked, because early detection saves lives. Find a qualified doctor, someone you feel comfortable with, someone who cares.

And last but not least, pray for God to help you. He will give you the strength to go through the many phases of breast cancer and above all, trust God with your life,

"He is the One who goes with you. He will not leave you nor forsake you" (Deut. 31:8, NKJV).

There is a song that I love, because it is everything that I shared with you in this book. It is my prayer that it will also become your testimony:

> My life is in You Lord,
> My strength is in You Lord,
> My hope is in You Lord, in You, it is in You!
> I praise You in all of my life,
> I praise You in all of my strength.
> With all of my life,
> With all of my strength
> All my hope is in You!

Perhaps some of you do not know the Lord but you would like to, or maybe you would like to have a more personal relationship with the Lord and want to rededicate your life to Jesus, then ask the Lord, and pray:

> *Dear Heavenly Father, I believe that You died for my sins on the cross. I ask You to forgive me of my sin, come into my heart, and forgive me. I want to live for You, and I want to know You! In Jesus' name, amen!*

If you have prayed this prayer, let someone know, or you can reach me by email at attiedv@aol.com. Visit my Web site for books at www.attiedevries.com.

Notes

Chapter 1
1. Jeanne A. Dunn, "Ann Jillian: Hope Belongs At Home," *Possibility* magazine, Nov./Dec. 1989, 8.
2. Ibid.

Chapter 3
1. "Have Thine Own Way, Lord," public domain. Music by George Coles Stebbins, words by Adelaide Addison Pollard, 1907.

Chapter 4
1. Jeanne A. Dunn, "Ann Jillian: Hope Belongs At Home," *Possibility* magazine, Nov./Dec. 1939, 8.
2. Ibid.
3. Ibid.

Chapter 5
1. Corrie ten Boom, *The Hiding Place* (New York: Random House, Inc., 1982), 256.

Chapter 7

1. Susan Love and Karen Lindsey, *Dr. Susan Love's Breast Book*, 2nd ed. (New York: Addison-Wesley Publishing Company, 1995), 627.

2. Roberta Altman and Michael J. Sarg, MD, *The Cancer Dictionary* (New York: Facts on File, 1992), 334.

3. Web site: www.vivelledot.com, accessed December 1, 2006.

4. Lydia Komarnicky, MD, Anne Rosenberg, MD, and Marian Betancourt, *What to Do if You Get Breast Cancer* (New York: Little, Brown and Company, 1995), 223.

5. Ibid.

6. For more information see http://uscnorriscancer. usc.edu/clinical_trials/ (accessed Jan. 24, 2007).

7. Keven M. Kelly, MD., SonoCiné, Hill Breast Center. Pasadena, CA, interview with author.

8. Altman and Sarg, *The Cancer Dictionary*, 334.

9. Ibid.

10. Marilynn Marchione, "Study favors MRI for Finding Breast Tumors," *The Orange County Register*, July 29, 2004.

11. Ibid.

Chapter 8

1. "Trust and Obey," public domain. Music by Daniel Brink Towner, words by John H. Sammis, 1887.

2. "Praise God, from Whom All Blessings Flow," public domain. Music by Genevan Psalter, 1551; attributed to Louis Bourgeois. Words by Thomas Ken.

Chapter 9

1. "He Is Lord," public domain.

Chapter 11

1. Web site: www.helenkeller.org, accessed December
   1, 2006.
2. "Great Is Thy Faithfulness," public domain. Music
   by William Runyan, words by Thomas Obediah
   Chrisholm, 1923.

Helpful Reading

1. The Word of God
2. *Nothing to Fear* by Larry Burkett
3. *A Spiritual Journey* by Judy Aste
4. *A Different Kind of Miracle* by Emilie Barnes
5. *Dear God It Is Cancer* by William A. Fintel and Gerald R. Mc Dermott
6. *What to Do if You Get Breast Cancer* by Lycia Komarnicky, MD, and Anne Rosenberg, MD
7. *Principles of Neurology* by Maurice Victor and Allan Ropper
8. *Dr. Susan Love's Breast Book* by Susan M. Love, MD, with Karen Lindsey
9. *Cancer Battle Plan* by Anne E. Frahm with David J. Frahm

Additional Information from the Author

Cancer patients can fly free. Contact Bonnie Le Var, president of the Corporate Angel Network, Inc., at the patient toll free number (866) 328–1313. They will help cancer patients fly for free wherever they need to go for cancer treatments.

SonoCiné
Hill Breast Center
50 Alessandro Pl.
Pasadena, CA 91105
(626) 793–6141
www.sonocine.com

University of Southern California
Norris Comprehensive Cancer Center
1441 Eastlake Ave.
Los Angeles, CA 90033
(323) 865–3933
Referrals: (323) 865–3105
www.targittrial.com

To Contact the Author

attiedv@aol.com
www.attidevries.com